COMPLETE ON DIABETES

COOKBOOK AND MEAL PLAN

A 4-WEEK MEAL PLAN WITH 30 MINUTES DELICIOUS DIABETES RECIPES

©Peter Coleman

All rights reserved. No parts of this publication may be reproduced, stored in retrieval system, or transmitted in any form or by any means, electronic, mechanical, photocopying, recording, or otherwise, without the prior written permission of the author.

CONTENTS

Introduction 6
- WHAT IS THE CAUSES DIABETES? 8
- Diabetics Treatment 13
- Diabetes and diet 14
- Diabetes Diagnosis 16
- Blood Tests for Diabetes 17
- Diabetes Prevention 21
- 12 Ways To Avoid Getting Diabetes. 21
- DIABETES IN CHILDREN 25
- Symptoms In Children. 26
- Diagnosis 27
- Prevention 28

HEALTHY AND DELICIOUS RECIPES THAT CAN HELP PEOPLE WITH DIABETES. 29
- BLACKENED TILAPIA WITH ZUCCHINI NOODLES 30
- SHRIMP & CORN STIR-FRY 31
- CHILI STEAK & PEPPERS 32
- SAUSAGE-TOPPED WHITE PIZZA. 33
- SPINACH AND MUSHROOM SMOTHERED CHICKEN 35
- FETA GARBANZO BEAN SALAD 36
- LEMON SALMON WITH BASIL 37
- FLAVORFUL GRILLED PORK TENDERLOIN. 38

ASPARAGUS TURKEY STIR-FRY	39
CHICKEN & VEGETABLE KABOBS	41
ASIAN LETTUCE WRAPS	42
COD AND ASPARAGUS BAKE	43
CHICKEN THIGHS WITH SHALLOTS & SPINACH	44
BALSAMIC CHICKEN WITH ROASTED TOMATOES	45
BEEF & SPINACH LO MEIN	46
BROILED COD	48
MEDITERRANEAN PORK AND ORZO	49
SAUSAGE ZUCCHINI SKILLET	50
CASHEW CHICKEN WITH GINGER	52
GREEN PEPPER STEAK	53
TORTILLA PIE	54
PORK & POTATO SUPPER	56
BALSAMIC-GLAZED BEEF SKEWERS	57
CHICKEN & GARLIC WITH FRESH HERBS	58
SKILLET SEA SCALLOPS	60
CHICKEN SAUSAGES WITH PEPPERS	61
CRUNCHY OVEN-BAKED TILAPIA	62
IN-A-PINCH CHICKEN & SPINACH	63
SKILLET BEEF AND POTATOES	64
CHICKEN VEGGIE PACKETS	65
POACHED EGGS WITH TARRAGON ASPARAGUS	66
SEASONED TILAPIA FILLETS	69

CHICKEN VEGGIE SKILLET	70
BAKED COD PICCATA WITH ASPARAGUS	72
STIR-FRY RICE BOWL	73
PEPPER STEAK WITH SQUASH	75
CURRY TURKEY STIR-FRY	76
MEDITERRANEAN TILAPIA	78
ROSEMARY GARLIC SHRIMP	79
STUFFED-OLIVE COD	80
LEMON-PEPPER TILAPIA WITH MUSHROOMS	81
CHICKEN SAUSAGES WITH POLENTA	83
SALMON WITH SPINACH & WHITE BEANS	84
GINGER VEGGIE BROWN RICE PASTA	85
SPICY TURKEY LETTUCE WRAPS	87
SPICED SALMON	88
CHICKEN & GOAT CHEESE SKILLET	89
GARLIC-MUSHROOM TURKEY SLICES	90
GRILLED CHICKEN CHOPPED SALAD	92
NAKED FISH TACOS	93
TILAPIA WITH CITRUS SAUCE	94
CHICKEN WITH FIRE-ROASTED TOMATOES	96
COD WITH BACON & BALSAMIC TOMATOES	97
CILANTRO LIME SHRIMP	99
CRUNCHY TUNA SALAD WITH TOMATOES	100
PEPPERED TUNA KABOBS	101

CHICKEN & SPANISH CAULIFLOWER "RICE" 102

CHERRY-CHICKEN LETTUCE WRAPS 104

PEPPER AND SALSA COD 105

SIMPLE GRILLED STEAK FAJITAS 106

TURKEY VERDE LETTUCE WRAPS.................................. 108

GARLIC TILAPIA WITH SPICY KALE 109

GRILLED CHICKEN AND MANGO SKEWERS 110

INTRODUCTION

Diabetes mellitus, or diabetes is a metabolic condition characterized by excessive blood sugar levels. Insulin transports sugar from the bloodstream into your cells, where it is stored or used for energy, your body either doesn't generate enough insulin or can't use the insulin it does make efficiently if you have diabetes. Diabetes can harm your nerves, eyes, kidneys, and other organs if left untreated.

Diabetes is divided into several types:

Diabetes type 1 is an autoimmune illness. In the pancreas, where insulin is produced, the immune system attacks and destroys cells It is unknown what is causing this attack, this kind of diabetes affects about 10% of diabetics, when your body develops resistant to insulin, sugar builds up in your blood resulting in type 2 diabetes.

High blood sugar in the course of pregnancy is known as gestational diabetes. This kind of diabetes is caused by the placenta's production of insulin-blocking substances although it has a similar name, diabetes insipidus is an uncommon illness that is unrelated to diabetes mellitus. It's a condition in which your kidneys excrete too much fluid from your body.

What are the many kinds of diabetes?

Diabetes is a collection of disorders in which the body does not make enough or any insulin, or does not use the insulin it does generate properly, or a combination of the two. When one or more of these events occurs, the body is unable to transport sugar from the blood into the cells, resulting in high blood sugar levels. One of your main energy sources is glucose, a type of sugar found in your blood. Sugar builds up in your blood due to a lack of insulin or insulin resistance. This can result in a variety of health issues.

The three main types of diabetes are:

- Type 1 diabetes
- Type 2 diabetes
- Gestational diabetes

Diabetes type 1 is autoimmune illness. In the pancreas, where insulin is produced, the immune system attacks and destroys cells, it is unknown what is causing this attack, this kind of diabetes affects about 10% of diabetics. When your body develops resistant to insulin, sugar builds up in your blood, resulting in type 2 diabetes. High blood sugar in the course of pregnancy is known as gestational diabetes insulin-blocking medications

WHAT IS THE CAUSES DIABETES?

Diabetes type 1

Diabetes type 1 is thought to be caused by an autoimmune disorder. This occurs when your immune system targets and destroys the insulin-producing beta cells in your pancreas. It is irreversible.

It is unclear what causes the attacks. Both hereditary and environmental factors could be to blame. It isn't assumed that lifestyle variables play a part.

Diabetes type 2

Insulin resistance is the first symptom of type 2 diabetes. This indicates that your body is unable to utilize insulin effectively. Your pancreas is stimulated to generate more insulin until it can no longer meet demand. Insulin production declines, resulting in elevated blood sugar levels.

Type 2 diabetes has an enigmatic cause. Among the possible contributors are:

- Genetics
- Physical inactivity
- Obesity

Other health and environmental variables could also be involved.

Diabetes Gestational: Insulin-blocking hormones released during pregnancy are responsible for gestational diabetes. During pregnancy, this kind of diabetes exclusively develops.

WHAT ARE THE SYMPTOMS?

The following are some of the most common diabetic symptoms:

- Excessive hunger and thirst
- Urination on a regular basis
- Drowsiness or exhaustion
- Itchy, dry skin
- Vision is blurry.
- Wounds that take a long time to heal.
- Dark patches of skin in the armpits and neck folds can be a sign of type 2 diabetes.

Type 2 diabetes takes longer to diagnose, you may have symptoms such as pain or numbness in your feet at the time of diagnosis.

Type 1 diabetes develops more quickly and might result in symptoms such as weight loss or diabetic ketoacidosis. When your blood sugar levels are extremely high but your body has little or no insulin, diabetic ketoacidosis can develop.

Symptoms in Men

Men with diabetes may experience diminished sex drive, erectile dysfunction (ED), and muscle weakness, in addition to the normal symptoms of the disease.

Symptoms in Women

Urinary tract infections, yeast infections, and dry, itchy skin are all signs of diabetes in women

Generally.

Both types of diabetes can cause symptoms at any age, but type 1 diabetes is more common in children and young people. Type 2 diabetes is found in persons over the age of 45. However, due to sedentary lifestyles and weight gain, type 2 diabetes is becoming more common among young people.

Type 1 diabetes can cause a variety of symptoms, including:

- Extreme hunger
- An increase in thirst
- Weight reduction that is unintentional
- urinating on a regular basis
- Vision that is blurry
- drowsiness
- It could also affect your moods.

Type 2 diabetes symptoms include:

- An increase in hunger
- An increase in thirst
- frequent Urination
- Vision that is blurred
- drowsiness
- Slow-healing sores

It's also possible that it'll lead to recurrent infections. This is due to the fact that high glucose levels make it difficult for the body to mend.

Gestational Diabetes

The majority of women with gestational diabetes experience no symptoms. Between the 24th and 28th weeks of pregnancy, a standard blood sugar test or oral glucose tolerance test is commonly conducted to detect the condition. A woman with gestational diabetes may experience increased thirst or urination in rare situations.

Generally.

Diabetic symptoms might be subtle at first, making them difficult to detect

DIABETES COMPLICATIONS

Blood sugar levels that are too high harm organs and tissues all over the body. The longer you live with high blood sugar, the more likely you are to have issues.

Diabetes has a number of complications, including:

- Heart disease, heart attack, and stroke are all conditions that can lead to death.
- Neuropathy is a condition that affects the nervous
- Nephropathy is a disease of the kidneys.
- Retinopathy is a condition that causes visual loss.
- Hearing loss
- Infections and non-healing ulcers on the feet are examples of foot injury skin conditions example bacterial and fungal infections
- Depression
- Dementia

Diabetics Treatment

Doctors use a variety of drugs to treat diabetes. Some of these medications are taken orally, while others are administered as injections.

Diabetic type 1 is a

Insulin is the most common type 1 diabetes treatment. It takes the place of a hormone that your body is unable to manufacture.

Insulin comes in four different forms. They differ in terms of how quickly they get to work and how long their effect last, which are:

Rapid-acting insulin kicks in within 15 minutes and has a 3- to 4-hour duration of action.

Short-acting insulin kicks in after 30 minutes and lasts for 6 to 8 hours.

Intermediate-acting insulin takes 1 to 2 hours to start working and lasts 12 to 18 hours.

Long-acting insulin kicks in a few hours after injection and lasts for at least 24 hours.

Type 2 diabetes

Your doctor will tell you how often you should check your blood glucose levels and you can properly manage type 2 diabetes. The objective is to stay within a certain range, some patients with type 2 diabetes can benefit from a healthy diet and regular exercise. If lifestyle changes aren't enough to control your blood sugar, you will need to take medication, the majority of type 2 diabetes treatments are taken orally. A handful are available as injections, however. Insulin may be necessary for certain patients with type 2 diabetes.

Diabetes and diet

The importance of good nutrition in diabetes management cannot be overstated. In other circumstances, simply modifying your diet may be enough to bring the disease under control.

Diabetic type 1

The kind of meals you eat affect your blood sugar level. Blood sugar levels rise quickly after eating starchy or sugary foods. Protein and fat, on the other hand, generate more gradual increases. Your doctor may advise you to restrict your daily carbohydrate intake. You'll also have to keep your carb intake in line with your insulin dosages. Consult a dietician for assistance in developing a diabetes food plan. Controlling your blood sugar can be as simple as eating the appropriate combination of protein, fat, and carbohydrates. Take a look at this advice to getting started on a type 1 diabetic diet.

Diabetes type 2

Eating the appropriate foods can help you lose weight while also controlling your blood sugar.

Carbohydrate counting is an important aspect of type 2 diabetic diet. A nutritionist can assist you in determining how many grams of carbohydrates you should consume at each meal.

Try to consume modest meals throughout the day to keep your blood sugar levels stable. Healthy foods to emphasize include:

- Fruits & Vegetables
- Fruits and vegetables
- Grain (whole)
- Poultry and fish are good sources of lean protein.
- Olive oil and nuts are good sources of healthy fats.

Other foods can jeopardize your efforts to keep your blood sugar under control. If you have diabetes, learn which foods you should avoid.

Gestational diabetes

During these nine months, it's critical for both you and your kid to eat a well-balanced diet. Choosing the appropriate foods can also help you avoid having to take diabetes medication.

Limit sugary and salty foods, and watch your portion sizes. You need some sugar to feed your growing kid, but you shouldn't eat too much of it.

Consider working with a dietitian or nutritionist to create an eating plan. They'll make sure your diet has the appropriate macronutrient balance.

Diabetes Diagnosis

Anyone who has diabetic symptoms or is at risk of developing the disease should be checked. During the second or third trimester of pregnancy, women are frequently screened for gestational diabetes.

These blood tests are used by doctors to determine prediabetes and diabetes.

After an 8-hour fast, the fasting plasma glucose (FPG) test checks your blood sugar.

The A1C test gives you a snapshot of your blood sugar levels for the last three months.

Between the 24th and 28th weeks of your pregnancy, your doctor will test your blood sugar levels to diagnose gestational diabetes.

Your blood sugar is examined one hour after you drink a sugary liquid during the glucose challenge test. The sooner you receive a diabetes diagnosis, the sooner you can begin treatment.

Who should be tested for diabetes?

Diabetes may or may not cause numerous symptoms in its early stages. If you have any of the early signs listed below, you should have your blood checked.

- Feeling constantly fatigued despite being exceedingly thirsty
- Even after eating, still hungry
- Vision that is hazy
- Urinating more frequently than normal.

- Having persistent sores or wounds

Even if they don't have any symptoms, some people should be checked for diabetes. If you're overweight (BMI greater than 25) and fall into any of the following criteria, the American Diabetes Association (ADA) recommends that you get tested for diabetes. You belong to a high-risk ethnic group (African-American, Latino, Native American, Pacific Islander, Asian-American, among others).

You have heart disease, high blood pressure, high triglycerides, low HDL cholesterol, or both.

You have a history of diabetes in your family.

You have a family history of high blood sugar or evidence of insulin resistance.

When you don't get enough exercise on a regular basis.

You have a history of gestational diabetes or polycystic ovarian syndrome (PCOS). If you're over 45, the American Diabetes Association also suggests getting a blood sugar test. This aids in the establishment of a blood sugar baseline. Because your risk of acquiring diabetes grows as you get older, testing can help you figure out if you're at risk.

Blood Tests for Diabetes

The A1c test measures how much sugar is in your blood.

A doctor can use blood tests to evaluate blood sugar levels in the body. The A1c test is one of the most popular because it provides an indication of blood sugar levels over time without requiring you to fast.

The glycated hemoglobin test is another name for the test. It determines how much glucose has bonded to red blood cells in your body over the previous two to three months because red blood cells have a three-month lifespan, the A1c test examines your average blood sugar for three months. Only a small volume of blood is needed for the test. The outcome is expressed as a percentage:

A score of fewer than 5.7 percent is considered normal.

Prediabetes is diagnosed when the results are between 5.7 and 6.4 percent.

Diabetes is diagnosed when the results are equal to or greater than 6.5 percent.

Only tests approved by the National Institute of Diabetes and Digestive and Kidney Diseases (NIDDKD) should be considered decisive enough to diagnose diabetes, according to the NGSP.

The A1c test may yield different results for different persons. This includes women who are pregnant or who have a hemoglobin variation that causes the test results to be erroneous. In some cases, your doctor may recommend a different type of diabetes test.

Blood sugar test at random

A random blood sugar test draws blood at any moment, regardless of when you last ate. Diabetes is diagnosed when the results are equal to or greater than 200 mg/dL.

Blood sugar levels after a fast

Blood is drawn after you've fasted overnight, which typically implies not eating for 8 to 12 hours:

It is usual to have a result of less than 100 mg/dL.

Prediabetes is indicated by results of 100 to 125 mg/dL.

Diabetes is diagnosed when the blood sugar level is 126 mg/dL or above after two tests.

Tolerance test for oral glucose

Over the course of two hours, the oral glucose test (OGTT) is performed. Your blood sugar is checked first, and then a sweet drink is administered. Your blood sugar levels are checked once more after two hours:

It is usual to have a result of less than 140 mg/dL.

Prediabetes is indicated by results of 140 to 199 mg/dL.

Diabetes is defined as a blood sugar level of 200 mg/dL or above.

Diabetic urine screening

To diagnose diabetes, urine tests are always done. If your doctor suspects you have type 1 diabetes, they'll likely utilize them. When adipose tissue is used as fuel instead of blood sugar, the body creates ketone bodies, these ketone bodies can be detected in urine by labs.

If you have moderate to high levels of ketone bodies in your urine, it could mean your body isn't producing enough insulin.

Gestational diabetes tests

When a woman is pregnant, she may develop gestational diabetes. The American Diabetes Association recommends that women with risk factors be tested for diabetes during their first appointment to see if they already have the disease. Gestational diabetes develops throughout the second and third trimesters of pregnancy.

To detect gestational diabetes, doctors may perform one of two tests. An initial glucose challenge test is the first step, a glucose syrup solution is consumed during this test. After an hour, blood is collected to check blood sugar levels, a blood sugar level of 130 to 140 mg/dL is considered normal, reading that is greater than typical suggests that more testing is required. Following up on the glucose tolerance testing, you won't be able to consume anything for the next 24 hours. A preliminary blood sugar level is determined, the expecting mother then consumes a high-sugar beverage. After that, the blood sugar is monitored every three hours. The results indicate gestational diabetes if a woman has two or more higher-than-normal values.

A two-hour glucose tolerance test, similar to the one described above, is performed in the second test. With this test, one out-of-range number would be diagnostic for gestational diabetes.

Diabetes Prevention

Because it is caused by an immune system dysfunction, type 1 diabetes cannot be prevented. You have no control over some factors of type 2 diabetes, such as your genes or your age.

Many additional diabetes risk factors, on the other hand, are within our power to influence. The majority of diabetes prevention methods entail making minor dietary and exercise changes.

Here are some things you can do if you've been diagnosed with prediabetes to delay or prevent type 2 diabetes:

A minimum of 150 minutes of cardiovascular exercise each week, such as walking or cycling is recommended.

Reduce the amount of saturated and trans fats in your diet, as well as refined carbs.

Fruits, vegetables, and whole grains should all be consumed in greater quantities.

Reduce the size of your meals.

If you're overweight or obese, your goal should be to reduce 7% of your body weight.

12 Ways To Avoid Getting Diabetes.
Sugar and refined carbs should be avoided in your diet.

Sugary diets and processed carbohydrates can put people at risk for diabetes on the fast track.

These foods are quickly broken down into little sugar molecules by your body and absorbed into your bloodstream.

Your pancreas is stimulated to generate insulin, a hormone that helps sugar go out of the bloodstream and into your body's cells, as a result of the spike in blood sugar.

Exercise on a regular basis.

Regular physical activity may aid in the prevention of diabetes. Your cells' insulin sensitivity will improve as a result of exercise. As a result, when you exercise, you need less insulin to keep your blood sugar levels in check.

As a primary beverage, drink water.

Water is without a doubt the most natural beverage available.

Furthermore, drinking mostly water helps you avoid beverages heavy in sugar, preservatives, and other potentially harmful substances.

If you are overweight or obese, you should lose weight.

Although type 2 diabetes does not affect everyone, it does affect the majority of people who develop it

Furthermore, those with prediabetes are more likely to carry extra weight around their waist and abdominal organs such as the liver, visceral fat is what it's called.

Stop Smoking

Heart disease, emphysema, and malignancies of the lungs, breast, prostate, and digestive tract have all been linked to smoking.

Smoking increased the risk of diabetes by 44 percent in ordinary smokers and 61 percent in persons who smoked more than 20 cigarettes per day, according to a review of numerous studies involving over million participants.

Maintain a Low-Carbohydrate Diet

Diabetes can be avoided by eating a ketogenic or very low-carb diet.

Although there are a variety of diets that can help you lose weight, very-low-carb diets have a lot of support. Your blood sugar levels will not rise as much if you limit your carb consumption as a result, your body requires less insulin to keep your blood sugar at a safe level.

Vitamin D Levels Should Be Optimized.

Vitamin D is important for blood sugar control. In fact, studies have shown that people who don't get enough vitamin D or have low blood levels of vitamin D have a higher risk of all types of diabetes. Most health organizations recommend a vitamin D blood level of at least 30 ng/ml (75 nmol/l).

Children who took vitamin D supplements had a 78 percent decreased chance of developing type 1 diabetes than children who did not get enough vitamin D.

The number of processed foods you eat should be reduced.

Minimizing your intake of processed foods is an obvious step you can take to improve your health.

They've been linked to everything from heart disease to obesity to diabetes.

Coffee or Tea

Although water should be your primary beverage, studies show that incorporating coffee or tea in your diet can help you avoid diabetes.

According to studies, drinking coffee on a regular basis lowers the risk of type 2 diabetes by 8–54 percent, with the biggest effect shown in those that are consume the most

Sedentary Behaviors Should Be Avoided

If you wish to avoid diabetes, you should avoid being sedentary.

You lead a sedentary lifestyle if you get little or very little physical activity and spend the majority of your day sitting.

Keep eyes on portion sizes.

Whether or not you choose to follow a low-carb diet, it's critical to avoid eating excessive amounts of food to lower your diabetes risk, especially if you're overweight.

In persons at risk of diabetes, eating too much food at once has been linked to higher blood sugar and insulin levels.

DIABETES IN CHILDREN

Type 1 and type 2 diabetes can affect children. Blood sugar control is especially crucial in young individuals because diabetes can harm vital organs like the heart and kidneys.

Type 1 diabetes

Diabetes with an autoimmune component frequently begins in childhood. Increased urination is one of the most common symptoms. After being toilet trained, children with type 1 diabetes may begin to wet the bed.

Extreme thirst, exhaustion, and hunger are also symptoms of the illness. It's critical that children with type 1 diabetes receive treatment as soon as possible. High blood sugar and dehydration are two medical crises that can occur as a result of the condition.

Diabetes type 2

Because type 2 diabetes is so uncommon in children, type 1 diabetes was once referred to as "juvenile diabetes." Type 2 diabetes is becoming more common in this age group as more youngsters become overweight or obese.

Type 2 diabetes, if left untreated, can lead to life-threatening complications such as heart disease, kidney failure, and blindness. Healthy food and exercise can assist your child in controlling their blood sugar levels and avoiding these issues.

Young people are more likely than ever to have type 2 diabetes.

Diabetes with an autoimmune component frequently begins in childhood. Increased urination is one of the most common symptoms. After being toilet trained, children with type 1 diabetes may begin to wet the bed.

Extreme thirst, exhaustion, and hunger are also symptoms of the illness. It's critical that children with type 1 diabetes receive treatment as soon as possible. High blood sugar and dehydration are two medical crises that can occur as a result of the condition

Symptoms In Children.
Children, teenagers, and adults all have diabetes symptoms that are comparable. While both types of diabetes share similar symptoms, there are certain distinctions that can help distinguish them.

Type 1 diabetes symptoms in children usually appear quickly and last only a few weeks. Symptoms of type 2 diabetes appear later. A diagnosis could take weeks, months, or even years to come.

Prior to receiving a diagnosis, weight loss is a common symptom. Infections with yeast might be a sign of diabetes in women.

Diabetic ketoacidosis (DKA) may be present at the time of diagnosis for certain persons. Because of a lack of insulin, the body begins to burn fat for energy. This is a serious condition that requires treatment.

People who recognize the four basic signs of type 1 diabetes may be able to acquire a diagnosis before DKA occurs.

People should be aware of the "4 Ts" in youngsters, according to Diabetes U.K.

Toilet: The youngster may be frequenting the bathroom, newborns may be wearing bulkier diapers, or bedwetting may be occurring after a period of being dry.

Thirsty: The child may be drinking more water than usual yet is still thirsty.

Fatigued: The child may be tired in a different way than normal.

Thinner: It's possible when the child is losing weight.

Diagnosis

Any youngster who exhibits signs or symptoms of diabetes should be screened by a physician. A urine test to look for sugar in the pee or a finger-prick blood test to assess the child's glucose levels are examples of this.

Children should be tested for diabetes, according to the National Institute for Health Care and Excellence, if they:

Have a history of type 2 diabetes in your family?

Have been diagnosed with obesity.

Acanthosis nigricans, for example, is a sign of insulin resistance.

Early detection improves the results for children with type 1 or type 2 diabetes.

Prevention

Type 1 diabetes cannot be prevented at this time, while type 2 diabetes is mostly preventable.

The following steps can assist in the prevention of type 2 diabetes in children:

Keep your weight in a healthy range: Obesity raises the risk of type 2 diabetes by increasing insulin resistance.

Maintain a healthy level of physical activity: Maintaining a healthy level of physical activity improves insulin resistance and aids with blood pressure management.

Limit sugary foods and beverages: Eating a lot of sugary foods can contribute to weight gain and insulin issues. Type 2 diabetes can be prevented by eating well-balanced, nutrient-dense diet rich in vitamins, fiber, and lean proteins.

Summary

Childhood and adolescent diabetes are becoming more common. Young individuals are far more likely to get type 1 diabetes than type 2 diabetes, yet both are on the rise.

A healthy diet, frequent exercise, and medications may usually manage the symptoms of both type 1 and type 2 diabetes. If you're at risk, get your blood sugar checked and follow your doctor's blood sugar management

HEALTHY AND DELICIOUS RECIPES THAT CAN HELP PEOPLE WITH DIABETES.

If one of your goals is to cook healthier at home in order to maintain good health condition on diabetes, then you will be prepared for success. The key part is to ensure that you have a large number of delicious new healthy recipes. It can be very painful to mix some nutritious and delicious things together. But once you have a meal plan your eating game will improve. In addition, if you have prepared a delicious and diabetes friendly meal and are ready, you will not want to order takeaway food.

It doesn't have to take a long time to prepare a dinner that is both healthy for diabetics and delicious for everyone. These simple diabetic meals take 30 minutes or less to prepare.

BLACKENED TILAPIA WITH ZUCCHINI NOODLES

Ingredients

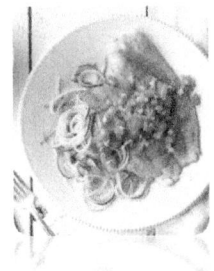

- 2 large zucchinis (about 1-1/2 pounds)
- 1-1/2 tsp ground cumin
- 1 cup Pico de Gallo
- 4 tilapia fillets (6 ounces each)
- ¾ tsp salt, divided
- ½ tsp pepper
- 2 tsp of olive oil
- 2 garlic cloves, minced
- ¼ tsp garlic powder
- ½ tsp smoked paprika

Directions

1. Trim the zucchini's ends and cut zucchini into thin strands with a spiralizer.
2. Combine cumin, ½ teaspoon salt, smoked paprika, pepper, and garlic powder; season both sides of tilapia generously. Heat the oil in a large nonstick skillet over medium-high heat. Cook tilapia in batches until it just begins to flake easily with a fork, about 2-3 minutes per side remove from the pan and set aside to keep heated.
3. In the same pan, cook zucchini and garlic over medium-high heat, tossing constantly with tongs, until slightly softened, about 1-2 minutes (do not overcook) then season with the remaining salt with tilapia and Pico de Gallo on the side.

Nutrition Facts

1 serving: 173 calories, 4g fat (1g saturated fat), 83mg cholesterol, 532mg sodium, 7g carbohydrate (5g sugars, 2g fiber), 32g protein.

SHRIMP & CORN STIR-FRY

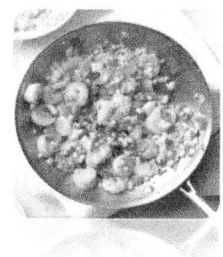

Ingredients

- 2 tsp olive oil
- 4 garlic cloves, minced
- 1 small onion, chopped
- ¼ tsp pepper
- 1-1/2 cups fresh or frozen corn, thawed
- 1 cup chopped tomatoes
- ½ tsp salt
- 2 small yellow summer squash, sliced
- 1-pound uncooked shrimp (26-30 per pound), peeled and deveined
- Hot cooked brown rice, optional
- ¼ tsp crushed red pepper flakes, optional
- ¼ cup chopped fresh basil

Directions

1. Heat the oil in a large skillet over medium-high heat. Stir the squash and onion for 2-3 minutes, or until the squash is crisp-tender.

2. Stir in the remaining 6 ingredients, as well as the pepper flakes if using, until the shrimp turn pink, about 3-4 minutes. Garnish with basil. If preferred, serve with rice

Nutrition Facts

1 serving (calculated without rice): 228 calories, 7g fat (1g saturated fat), 124mg cholesterol, 332mg sodium, 19g carbohydrate (8g sugars, 3g fiber), 23g protein.

CHILI STEAK & PEPPERS

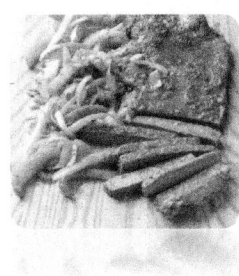

Ingredients:

- 1 tsp lime juice
- 1 tsp brown sugar
- 2 tsp chili sauce
- ½ tsp salt, divided
- 1 medium onion, halved and sliced
- 1 medium sweet yellow pepper, cut into strips
- 2 tsp olive oil
- 1 small garlic clove, minced
- 1 beef top sirloin steak (1-1/4 pounds)
- 1 medium green pepper, cut into strips
- 1/8 tsp pepper
- ¼ cup reduced-fat sour cream
- 1 teaspoon prepared horseradish
- ½ tsp crushed red pepper flakes

Directions

1. Brush the steak with a mixture of chili sauce, lime juice, brown sugar, pepper flakes, and 1/4 teaspoon salt. Broil steaks 4-6 inches from the heat for 5-7 minutes on each side or until desired doneness is achieved (a thermometer should read 135° for medium-rare, 140° for medium, and 145° for medium-well).

2. Meanwhile, sauté onion, green and yellow peppers, and garlic in oil in a large skillet until tender. Cook for 1 minute more after adding the garlic, pepper, and remaining salt. Mix sour cream and horseradish in a small bowl. Steak should be sliced and served with the pepper combination and sauce.

Nutrition Facts

4 ounces cooked beef with 1/3 cup pepper mixture and 1 tablespoon sauce: 165 calories, 7g fat (3g saturated fat), 62mg cholesterol, 345mg sodium, 10g carbohydrate (8g sugars, 2g fiber), 32g protein.

SAUSAGE-TOPPED WHITE PIZZA.

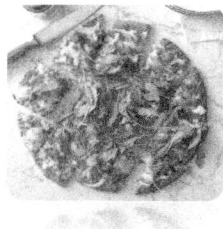

Ingredients:

- 2 hot Italian turkey sausage links, casings removed

- ¼ tsp garlic powder
- ½ cup shredded part-skim mozzarella cheese
- 1 small onion, halved and thinly sliced
- 1 cup reduced-fat ricotta cheese
- 1 prebaked 12-inch thin whole wheat pizza crust
- ½ tsp Italian seasoning
- 1 medium sweet red pepper, julienned
- ¼ tsp freshly ground pepper
- ¼ tsp crushed red pepper flakes, optional
- 2 cups arugula or baby spinach

Directions

1. Pre-heat the oven to 450 degrees Fahrenheit. Cook and shred sausage in a large skillet over medium-high heat until no longer pink, about 4-6 minutes. Combine ricotta cheese and garlic powder in a mixing bowl.
2. Spread the ricotta cheese mixture over the crust on a baking sheet. Sausage, red pepper, and onion are layered on top, followed by seasonings and mozzarella cheese.
3. Bake for 8-10 minutes on a lower oven rack, until the edge is lightly browned and the cheese is melted. Garnish with arugula

Nutrition Facts

1 slice: 235 calories, 5g fat (4g saturated fat), 20mg cholesterol, 405mg sodium, 26g carbohydrate (4g sugars, 4g fiber), 14g protein.

SPINACH AND MUSHROOM SMOTHERED CHICKEN

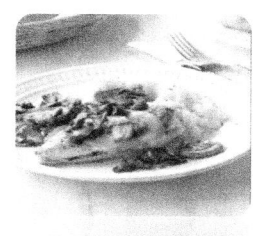

Ingredients:

- 1-1/2 tsp olive oil
- ½ tsp rotisserie chicken seasoning
- 1-3/4 cups sliced fresh mushrooms
- 4 boneless skinless chicken breast halves (4 ounces each)
- 2 tsp chopped pecans
- 3 green onions, sliced
- 2 slices reduced-fat provolone cheese, halved
- 3 cups fresh baby spinach

Directions

1. Prepare the grill or broiler by preheating it. Sauté mushrooms and green onions in a large skillet over medium-high heat until soft. Stir in the spinach and pecans until they're completely wilted. Keep warm by removing from the heat.

2. Season the chicken. 4-5 minutes per side, covered, on an oiled grill rack over medium heat or broil 4 inches from heat on a greased broiler pan until a

thermometer reads 165°. Grill or broil the cheese until it melts. Top with the mushroom mixture before serving.

Nutrition Facts

1 serving: 187 calories, 5g fat (2g saturated fat), 68mg cholesterol, 212mg sodium, 5g carbohydrate (1g sugars, 2g fiber), 26g protein.

FETA GARBANZO BEAN SALAD

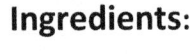

Ingredients:

- *5 cups torn mixed salad greens*
- 1 can (15 ounces) garbanzo beans or chickpeas, rinsed and drained
- 1 can (2-1/4 ounces) sliced ripe olives, drained
- 1 medium tomato, seeded and chopped
- 1/8 tsp pepper
- ¼ cup thinly sliced red onion

- 3 tsp olive oil
- 1-1/2 cups coarsely chopped English cucumber (about ½ medium)
- 1 tsp lemon juice
- ¼ cup chopped fresh parsley
- ½ cup crumbled feta cheese
- ¼ tsp salt

Directions

Place the 11 ingredients in a large bowl, toss properly then sprinkle with cheese.

Nutrition Facts

2 cups: 248 calories, 15g fat (3g saturated fat), 8mg cholesterol, 563mg sodium, 22g carbohydrate (4g sugars, 5g fiber), 8g protein.

LEMON SALMON WITH BASIL

Ingredients

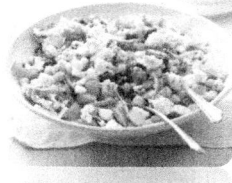

- ½ tsp salt
- ¼ tsp pepper
- 2 medium lemons, thinly sliced
- 1 tsp grated lemon zest
- 2 tsp thinly sliced fresh basil
- 2 tsp olive oil
- 4 salmon fillets (6 ounces each)

- Additional fresh basil

Directions

1. Pre-heat the oven to 375 degrees. In a greased 15x10x1-inch baking pan, place the salmon. Drizzle with oil, then season with lemon zest, salt, and pepper, as well as 2 tablespoons basil and lemon slices.
2. Bake for 15-20 minutes, or until the fish easily flakes with a fork. Add additional basil on top if desired.

Nutrition Facts.

1 salmon fillet: 234 calories, 15g fat (3g saturated fat), 65mg cholesterol, 341mg sodium, 3g carbohydrate (1g sugars, 1g fiber), 26g protein.

FLAVORFUL GRILLED PORK TENDERLOIN.

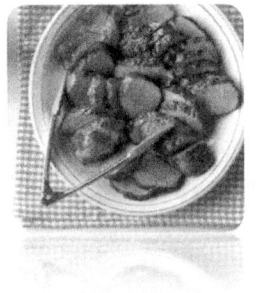

Ingredients

- ¾ tsp seasoned salt
- 2 pork tenderloins (1 pound each)
- ¾ tsp onion powder
- ¾ tsp garlic powder
- ¾ tsp chili powder
- ¾ tsp salt

- ¾ teaspoon poultry seasoning
- 1/8 tsp cayenne pepper

Directions

Seasonings should be mixed together and sprinkled over the tenderloins. Grill, covered, over medium heat for 20-25 minutes, or until thermometer reads 145°, flipping occasionally. Allow for a 5-minute rest before slicing.

Nutrition Facts.

3 ounces cooked pork: 114calories, 6g fat (1g saturated fat), 46mg cholesterol, 356mg sodium, 1g carbohydrate (0 sugars, 0 fiber), 25g protein.

ASPARAGUS TURKEY STIR-FRY

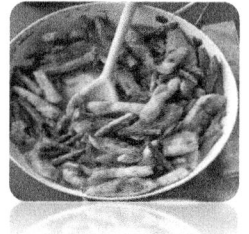

Ingredients:

- 1 pound turkey breast tenderloins, cut into ½-inch strips
- ¼ cup chicken broth
- 1 tsp lemon juice
- 1 jar (2 ounces) sliced pimientos, drained
- 2 tsp cornstarch
- 1-pound fresh asparagus, trimmed and cut into 1-1/2-inch pieces

- 1 tsp soy sauce
- 1 garlic clove, minced
- 2 tsp canola oil, divided

Directions

1. Whisk together the cornstarch, broth, lemon juice, and soy sauce in a small mixing bowl until smooth. Stir-fry the turkey and garlic in 1 tablespoon oil in a large skillet or wok until the flesh is no longer pink; remove from the skillet and keep warm.

2. Cook asparagus until crisp-tender in the remaining oil. Pimientos should be added at this point. Stir the broth mixture into the pan and simmer, stirring constantly, for 1 minute, or until it has thickened. Return the turkey to the pan and cook until it is fully cooked.

Nutrition Facts

1-1/2cups: 195 calories, 9g fat (1g saturated fat), 56mg cholesterol, 214mg sodium, 7g carbohydrate (1g sugars, 1g fiber), 25g protein.

CHICKEN & VEGETABLE KABOBS

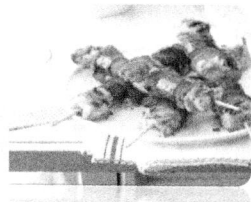

Ingredients

- 1 medium zucchini, cut into 1-1/2-inch pieces
- 1-pound boneless skinless chicken breasts, cut into 1-1/2-inch cubes
- 1 medium red onion, cut into thick wedges
- 2/3 cup sun-dried tomato salad dressing, divided
- 1 medium sweet red pepper, cut into 1-1/2-inch pieces

Directions

1. Combine the chicken and vegetables in a large mixing bowl. Drizzle 1/3 cup dressing over the salad and toss to coat. Thread chicken and vegetables alternately onto four metal or wet wooden skewers.

2. Cover and grill kabobs over medium heat or broil 4 inches from heat for 8-10 minutes, turning occasionally and basting with remaining dressing during the last 3 minutes

Nutrition Facts

1 kabob: 215 calories, 10g fat (1g saturated fat), 63mg cholesterol, 468mg sodium, 12g carbohydrate (7g sugars, 4g fiber), 24g protein.

ASIAN LETTUCE WRAPS

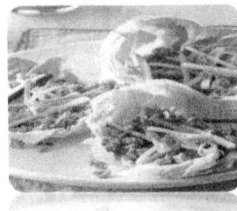

Ingredients

- 1 tsp canola oil
- 2 cups bean sprouts
- 1 medium carrot, julienned
- 1 jalapeno pepper, seeded and minced
- 1 tsp sugar or sugar substitute blend equivalent to 1 tablespoon sugar
- 2 green onions, thinly sliced
- 2 tsp minced fresh basil
- 2 garlic cloves, minced
- 1-pound lean ground turkey
- 2 tsp lime juice
- 2 tsp reduced-sodium soy sauce
- 12 Bibb or Boston lettuce leaves
- 1 medium cucumber, julienned
- 1 to 2 tsp chili garlic sauce

Directions

Heat the oil in a large skillet over medium heat. Cook for 6-8 minutes, or until turkey is no longer pink and crumbles easily. Cook for another 2 minutes after adding the jalapeño, green onions, and garlic. Heat through basil, lime juice, soy sauce, chili garlic sauce, and sugar.

To serve, stuff lettuce leaves with turkey mixture and cucumber, carrot, and bean sprouts. Fold the lettuce over the filling and tuck it in.

Nutrition Facts

3 lettuce wraps: 262 calories, 10g fat (3g saturated fat), 78mg cholesterol, 413mg sodium, 8g carbohydrate (5g sugars, 3g fiber), 23g protein.

COD AND ASPARAGUS BAKE

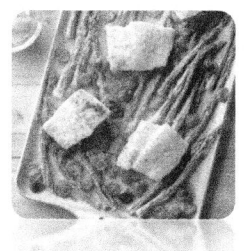

Ingredients

- 1&1/2 tsp grated lemon zest
- 1-pound fresh thin asparagus, trimmed
- 4 cod fillets (4 ounces each)
- ¼ cup grated Romano cheese
- 1 pint cherry tomatoes, halved
- 2 tsp lemon juice

Directions

1. Pre heat the oven to 375 degrees. Brush a 15x10x1-inch baking pan with oil and place the cod and asparagus in it. Toss in the tomatoes, cut sides down. Brush the fish with lemon juice and lemon zest. Romano cheese should be sprinkled over the fish and vegetables. Bake for about 12 minutes, or until the fish begins to flake easily with a fork.

2. Take the pan out of the oven and preheat the broiler. Broil cod mixture 3-4 inches from fire for 2-3 minutes, or until veggies are lightly browned.

Nutrition Facts

1 serving: 126 calories, 3g fat (2g saturated fat), 34mg cholesterol, 153mg sodium, 6g carbohydrate (4g sugars, 2g fiber), 26g protein.

CHICKEN THIGHS WITH SHALLOTS & SPINACH

Ingredients

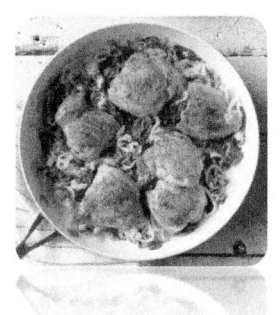

- ¼ cup reduced-fat sour cream
- 1-1/2 tsp olive oil
- 1/3 cup white wine or reduced-sodium chicken broth
- 4 shallots, thinly sliced
- ½ tsp pepper
- 6 boneless skinless chicken thighs (about 1-1/2 pounds)
- 1 package (10 ounces) fresh spinach, trimmed
- ½ tsp seasoned salt
- ¼ tsp salt

Directions

1. Season chicken with salt & pepper. Heat oil in a large nonstick skillet on a medium heat. Cook for 6

minutes on each side, or until a thermometer reads 170°. Remove from pan and set aside to keep heated.
2. Shallots should be cooked and stirred in the same pan until soft. Toss in the wine and bring to a boil. Cook until the wine has been reduced in half. Cook, stirring constantly, until the spinach is wilted. Add the sour cream and serve with the chicken.

Nutrition Facts

1 chicken thigh with ¼ cup spinach mixture: 245 calories, 10g fat (3g saturated fat), 75mg cholesterol, 326mg sodium, 8g carbohydrate (4g sugars, 1g fiber), 27g protein.

BALSAMIC CHICKEN WITH ROASTED TOMATOES

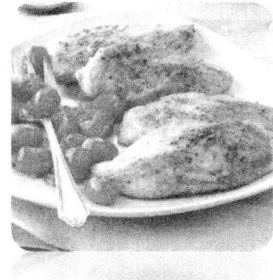

Ingredients

- 4 boneless skinless chicken breast halves (6 ounces each)
- 2 tsp olive oil, divided
- ½ tsp salt
- 2 tsp honey
- 2 tsp balsamic glaze
- 2 cups grape tomatoes
- ½ tsp pepper

Directions:

1. Pre heat the oven to 400 degrees. Mix 1 tablespoon oil and honey in a small bowl. Toss in the tomatoes and toss to coat, place the batter in a greased 15x10x1-inch baking pan. Bake for 5-7 minutes, or until the cheese has softened.
2. Using a meat mallet, pound chicken breasts to a thickness of ½inches; season with salt and pepper then heat the remaining oil in a large skillet on a medium-high heat. Cook for 5-6 minutes on each side, or until the chicken is no longer pink. Serve with roasted tomatoes and a glaze drizzled on top.

Nutrition Facts

1 chicken breast half with ½ cup tomatoes and 1-1/2 teaspoons glaze: 205 calories, 12g fat (2g saturated fat), 76mg cholesterol, 324mg sodium, 12g carbohydrate (12g sugars, 1g fiber), 32g protein.

BEEF & SPINACH LO MEIN

Ingredients

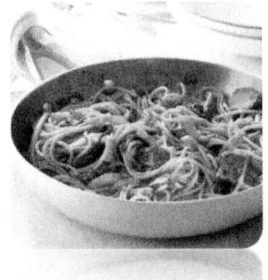

- ¼ cup hoisin sauce
- 2 tsp sesame oil
- 2 tsp soy sauce
- 1 tsp water

- 2 garlic cloves, minced
- ¼ tsp crushed red pepper flakes
- 6 ounces uncooked spaghetti
- 1 package (10 ounces) fresh spinach, coarsely chopped
- 2 green onions, sliced
- 4 tsp canola oil, divided
- 1 red chili pepper, seeded and thin
- 1 pound beef top round steak, thinly sliced
- 1 can (8 ounces) sliced water chestnuts, drained

Directions

1. Toss the first six ingredients together in a small mixing bowl. In a large mixing bowl, transfer 1/4 cup of the mixture; add the beef and stir to coat. Allow 10 minutes for the marinade to come to room temperature.
2. Follow the package directions for cooking spaghetti. 1 1/2 teaspoons canola oil, heated in a large skillet Stir-fry for 1-2 minutes, or until no longer pink, with half of the meat mixture. Taking it out of the pan Continue with the remaining beef mixture and 1-1/2 teaspoons oil.
3. In the remaining canola oil, cook the water chestnuts and green onions for 30 seconds. Cook until the spinach has wilted, then add the remaining hoisin mixture. Return the steak to the pan and cook until it is fully cooked
4. Drain the spaghetti and toss it with the beef mixture. Chili pepper should be sprinkled on top.

Nutrition Facts

1-1/3 cups: 234 calories, 10g fat (2g saturated fat), 51mg cholesterol, 225mg sodium, 35g carbohydrate (7g sugars, 4g fiber), 28g protein.

BROILED COD

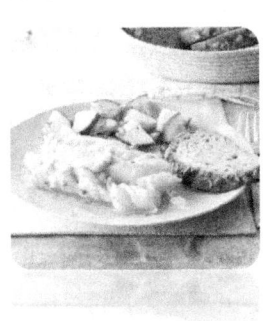

Ingredients

- ½ tsp sugar
- 2 tsp butter
- 1/8 tsp salt
- 1/8 tsp paprika
- 1/8 tsp pepper
- 2 cod fillets (6 ounces each)
- 1/8 tsp garlic powder
- 1/8 tsp curry powder
- ¼ cup fat-free Italian salad dressing

Directions:

1. Preheat the oven to broil. Mix first 7 ingredients in a small bowl; add cod and turn to coat. Allow for 10-15 minutes of resting time.

2. Place the fillets on a broiler pan's greased rack and discard the remaining marinade. Broil 3-4 inches from heat for 10-12 minutes, or until salmon just

begins to flake easily with a fork. Butter the top of the dish.

Nutrition Facts

1 fillet: 146 calories, 6g fat (4g saturated fat), 47mg cholesterol, 325mg sodium, 4g carbohydrate (2g sugars, 0 fiber), 23g protein.

Diabetic Exchanges: 4 lean meat, 1 fat.

MEDITERRANEAN PORK AND ORZO

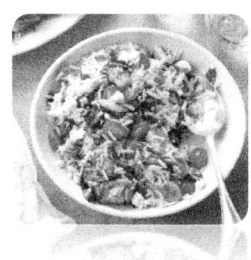

Ingredients

- 1-1/2 pounds pork tenderloin
- 1-1/4 cups uncooked orzo pasta
- 3 quarts water
- ¼ tsp salt
- 2 tsp olive oil
- ¾ cup crumbled feta cheese
- 1 package (6 ounces) fresh baby spinach
- 1 cup grape tomatoes, halved

- 1 tsp coarsely ground pepper

Directions:

1. Season the pork with pepper and cut it into 1-inch cubes. Heat the oil in a large nonstick skillet over medium heat. Cook and stir until the pork is no longer pink, about 8-10 minutes.
2. Meanwhile, bring water to a boil in a Dutch oven. Cook, uncovered, for 8 minutes after adding the orzo and salt. Stir in the spinach and heat for another 45-60 seconds, or until the orzo is cooked and the spinach has wilted. Drain.
3. Toss tomatoes into the pork and heat through. Combine the orzo and cheese in a mixing bowl.

Nutrition Facts

1-1/3 cups: 252 calories, 12g fat (5g saturated fat), 62mg cholesterol, 343mg sodium, 35g carbohydrate (3g sugars, 2g fiber), 34g protein. Diabetic Exchanges: 3 lean meat, 3 starch, 1 vegetable, 1 fat.

SAUSAGE ZUCCHINI SKILLET

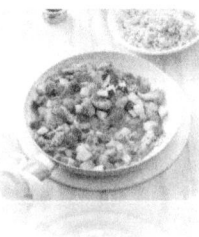

Ingredients

- 1-pound Italian turkey sausage links, casings removed
- 2 cups hot cooked brown rice
- 1 can (14-1/2 ounces) no-salt-added diced tomatoes, undrained

- 2 large zucchinis, cut into ½-in. pieces
- 2 garlic cloves, minced
- ¼ tsp pepper
- 1 large sweet onion, chopped

Directions.

1. Cook sausage, zucchini, and onion in a large nonstick skillet coated with cooking spray for 6-8 minutes, or till when sausage is no longer pink, breaking up sausage into crumbles. Cook for a further minute after adding the garlic. Drain.

2. Add the tomatoes and pepper to the pot and bring to a boil. Reduce heat to low and cook, stirring periodically, for 4-5 minutes, or until liquid has evaporated. Serve with rice.

Nutrition Facts

1-1/4 cups sausage mixture with ½ cup cooked rice: 252 calories, 5g fat (3g saturated fat), 42mg cholesterol, 463mg sodium, 33g carbohydrate (7g sugars, 3g fiber), 15g protein. Diabetic Exchanges: 2 lean meat, 2 vegetable, 1-1/2 starch.

CASHEW CHICKEN WITH GINGER

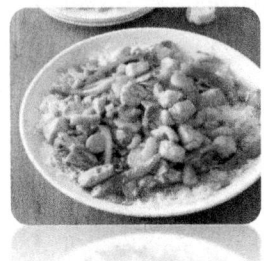

Ingredients

- 1 tsp brown sugar
- 1 small green pepper, cut into strips
- 1-1/4 cups chicken broth
- 2 tsp soy sauce
- Hot cooked rice
- ¾ cup salted cashews
- 2 tsp cornstarch
- 3 tsp canola oil, divided
- 4 green onions, sliced
- ½ pound sliced fresh mushrooms
- 1 can (8 ounces) sliced water chestnuts, drained
- 1-1/2 tsp grated fresh gingerroot
- 1-1/2 pounds boneless skinless chicken breasts, cut into 1-inch pieces

Directions

1. Whisk together the first four ingredients until its smooth.2 teaspoons oil, heated in a large skillet over medium-high heat; stir-fry chicken until no longer pinks. Remove the pan from the heat.
2. In the same pan, heat the remaining oil over medium-high heat and stir-fry the mushrooms, pepper, water chestnuts, and ginger for 3-5 minutes, or until the pepper is crisp-tender. Bring the broth mixture to a boil in the pan with the green

onions. Cook, stirring constantly, until the sauce has thickened, about 1-2 minutes.

3. Heat through the chicken and cashews. Serve with rice.

Nutrition Facts

¾ cup chicken mixture: 349 calories, 14g fat (3g saturated fat), 64mg cholesterol, 630mg sodium, 18g carbohydrate (6g sugars, 3g fiber), 28g protein. Diabetic Exchanges: 3 lean meat, 3 fat, 1 starch.

GREEN PEPPER STEAK

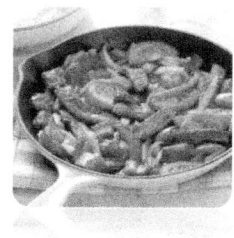

Ingredients

- 2 small onions, cut into thin wedges
- ¼ cup water
- 2 tsp canola oil, divided
- Hot cooked rice
- 1 medium green pepper, cut into 1-inch pieces
- 1 pound beef top sirloin steak, cut into ¼-in.-thick strips
- ¼ cup reduced-so dim soy sauce
- 1 tsp cornstarch
- 2 celery ribs, sliced diagonally

Directions

1. In a large mixing bowl, whisk together the cornstarch, soy sauce, and water until smooth. 1 tablespoon oil, heated in a large skillet over medium-high heat; stir-fry beef until browned, about 2-3 minutes. Remove the pan from the heat.

2. In the remaining oil, stir-fry the onions, celery, and pepper for 3 minutes. Combine cornstarch and water in a mixing bowl; add to pan. Bring to a boil, then cook and stir for 1-2 minutes, or until thickened and bubbling. Heat through the tomatoes and meat. Serve with rice.

Nutrition Facts

1 serving: 239 calories, 14g fat (2g saturated fat), 42mg cholesterol, 625mg sodium, 12g carbohydrate (4g sugars, 2g fiber), 26g protein. Diabetic Exchanges: 3 lean meat, 1 vegetable, 1-1/2 fat.

TORTILLA PIE

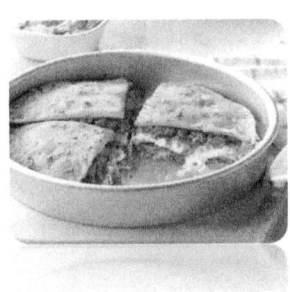

Ingredients

- ½ pound lean ground beef (90% lean)
- 1 can (14-1/2 ounces) Mexican diced tomatoes, drained
- ½ cup chopped onion
- 1 tsp chili powder

- 2 garlic cloves, minced
- ½ tsp ground cumin
- 4 whole wheat tortillas (8 inches)
- ¾ cup reduced-fat ricotta cheese
- ¼ cup shredded part-skim mozzarella cheese
- 3 tsp minced fresh cilantro, divided
- ½ cup shredded cheddar cheese

Directions:

1. Pre-heat the oven to 400 degrees. Cook and crumble beef with onion and garlic in a large skillet over medium heat until no longer pink, about 4-6 minutes. Toss in the tomatoes and seasonings. Bring to a boil, then turn off the heat. Combine ricotta cheese, mozzarella cheese, and 2 tablespoons cilantro in a small bowl.
2. Spray a 9-inch round baking pan with cooking spray and place 1 tortilla in it. Half of the meat sauce, 1 tortilla, ricotta mixture, another tortilla, and the remaining meat sauce are layered on top. Sprinkle the remaining cilantro and cheddar cheese on top of the remaining tortilla.
3. Bake for 15-20 minutes, covered, until thoroughly heated.

Nutrition Facts

1 serving: 326 calories, 12g fat (6g saturated fat), 46mg cholesterol, 436mg sodium, 26g carbohydrate (5g sugars, 5g fiber), 24g protein. Diabetic Exchanges: 2medium-fat meat, 2 starch.

PORK & POTATO SUPPER

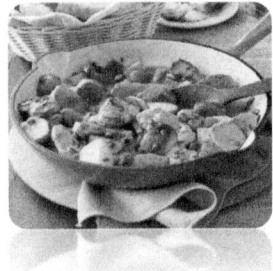

Ingredients

- 1 cup sliced fresh mushrooms
- 2 tsp all-purpose flour
- 4 green onions, sliced
- ¼ tsp pepper
- 2 tsp butter, divided
- 1 pork tenderloin (1 pound), cut into ¼-inch slices
- 8 small red potatoes, quartered
- 2 garlic cloves, minced
- 1 can (14-1/2 ounces) reduced-sodium chicken broth, divided
- 2 tsp Worcestershire sauce
- ¼ tsp salt

Directions

1. Melt 1 tablespoon of butter in a 12-inch skillet over medium-high heat. Cook for 2-4 minutes per side or until meat is cooked. Remove the pan from the oven.
2. dissolve the remaining butter in the same pan over medium-high heat. Cook, stirring constantly, until the mushrooms are almost soft. Cook for another minute after adding the garlic. Add the potatoes, 1 1/2 cups broth, Worcestershire sauce, salt, and pepper and mix well. Raise the heat to high and bring the water to a boil. Reduce heat to low and cook for 10-15 minutes, covered, until potatoes are cooked.

3. In a small mixing bowl, whisk together the flour and remaining broth until smooth. Add it to the mushroom mixture. Bring to a boil, then continue to cook and stir until the sauce has thickened then add the green onions and stir to combine. Return the meat to the pan and heat it all the way through.

Nutrition Facts

1-1/2 cups: 282 calories, 10g fat (5g saturated fat), 78mg cholesterol, 565mg sodium, 21g carbohydrate (2g sugars, 2g fiber), 27g protein. Diabetic Exchanges: 3 lean meat, 1-1/2 fat, 1 starch.

BALSAMIC-GLAZED BEEF SKEWERS

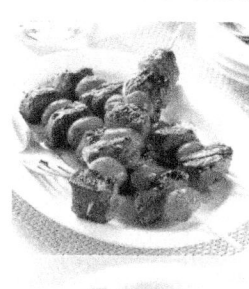

- **Ingredients**
- 1 tsp Dijon mustard
- 2 cups cherry tomatoes
- ¼ cup barbecue sauce
- 1 pound beef top sirloin steak, cut into 1-inch cubes
- ¼ cup balsamic vinaigrette

Directions

1. In a large mixing bowl, whisk together the vinaigrette, barbecue sauce, and mustard until well combined.1/4 cup of the mixture should be

saved for basting. Toss the remaining mixture with the steak and toss to coat.
2. Thread beef and tomatoes alternately onto four metal or soaked wooden skewers. Grill rack should be lightly greased.
3. Grill skewers, cover over medium heat for 6-9 minutes or until its desired doneness is reached, turning occasionally and basting frequently with reserved vinaigrette mixture during the last 3 minutes.

Nutrition Facts

1 skewer: 134 calories, 5g fat (2g saturated fat), 42mg cholesterol, 265mg sodium, 7g carbohydrate (5g sugars, 1g fiber), 24g protein. Diabetic Exchanges: 3 lean meat, 1-1/2 fat, ½ starch.

CHICKEN & GARLIC WITH FRESH HERBS

Ingredients

- 6 boneless skinless chicken thighs (about 1-1/2 pounds)
- ½ tsp salt
- 1 cup chicken stock
- 1 tsp minced fresh rosemary or ¼ teaspoon dried rosemary, crushed
- ¼ tsp pepper

- 1 tsp olive oil
- 2 tsp brandy or chicken stock
- 10 garlic cloves, peeled and halved
- ½ tsp minced fresh thyme or 1/8 teaspoon dried thyme
- 1 tsp minced fresh chives

Directions

1. Season chicken with salt and pepper before serving. Heat the oil in a big cast-iron pan or another heavy skillet over medium-high heat. Both sides of the chicken should be browned. Remove the pan from the heat.
2. Remove the skillet from the heat and add the garlic cloves, halved, and the brandy. Return to the fire and cook, stirring constantly, until the liquid has almost completely evaporated, about 1-2 minutes.
3. Return the chicken to the pan after adding the liquid, rosemary, and thyme. Let the water to boil. Reduce heat to low and cook, uncovered, for 6-8 minutes, or until a thermometer reads 170°. Sprinkle chives on top.

Nutrition Facts.

1 chicken thigh with 2 tablespoons cooking juices: 186 calories, 12g fat (3g saturated fat), 66mg cholesterol, 283mg sodium, 2g carbohydrate (0 sugars, 0 fiber), 23g protein. Diabetic Exchanges: 3 lean meat, ½ fat.

SKILLET SEA SCALLOPS

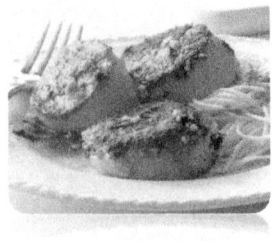

Ingredients

- ½ tsp salt
- 2 tsp lemon juice
- ¼ cup white wine or reduced-sodium chicken broth
- 2 tsp butter
- 1 tsp olive oil
- 1 pound sea scallops
- 1 garlic clove, minced
- ½ cup dry bread crumbs
- 1 tsp minced fresh parsley

Directions

1. Toss bread crumbs with salt in a small basin. Coat both sides of scallops with crumb mixture, patting to help coating adhere.
2. Dissolve the butter and oil in a large skillet over medium-high heat, Cook for 1 1/2 to 2 minutes per side, or until firm and opaque. Remove from pan and set aside to keep heated.
3. In the same pan, combine the wine, lemon juice, and garlic; bring to a boil. Add in the parsley and mix well. Drizzle over the scallops and serve right away.

Nutrition Facts

1 serving: 186 calories, 11g fat (4g saturated fat), 42mg cholesterol, 573mg sodium, 12g carbohydrate (1g sugars,

1g fiber), 24g protein. Diabetic Exchanges: 3 lean meat, 2 fat, 1 starch.

CHICKEN SAUSAGES WITH PEPPERS

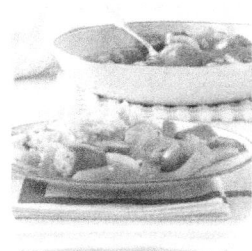

Ingredients

- 1 small onion, halved and sliced
- 1 tsp olive oil
- 1 package (12 ounces) fully cooked apple chicken sausage links or flavor of your choice, cut into 1-inch pieces
- 1 small sweet red pepper, julienned
- 1 small sweet orange pepper, julienned
- 1 garlic clove, minced

Directions

Sauté onion and peppers in oil in a large nonstick skillet until crisp-tender. Cook for a further minute after adding the garlic then add the sausages and heat thoroughly.

Nutrition Facts

1 cup: 175 calories, 13g fat (3g saturated fat), 54mg cholesterol, 353mg sodium, 13g carbohydrate (12g sugars, 1g fiber), 12g protein. Diabetic Exchanges: 3 lean meat, 1 vegetable, ½ starch, ½ fat.

CRUNCHY OVEN-BAKED TILAPIA

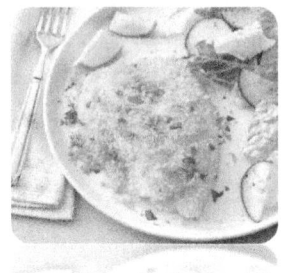

Ingredients

- 2 tsp minced fresh cilantro or parsley
- ½ tsp salt
- 1 tsp reduced-fat mayonnaise
- ¼ tsp pepper
- ¼ tsp grated lime zest
- 1 tsp lime juice
- 4 tilapia fillets (6 ounces each)
- ¼ tsp onion powder
- ½ cup panko bread crumbs
- Cooking spray

Directions

1. Pre heat the oven to 425 degrees. Spray a baking sheet with cooking spray and place the fillets on it. Mayonnaise, lime juice and zest, salt, onion powder, and pepper should all be combined in a small basin. Coat the fish in the mayonnaise mixture. Using a spritz of cooking spray, coat the bread crumbs.

2. Bake for 15-20 minutes, or until the fish easily flakes with a fork then add cilantro to the top.

Nutrition Facts

1 fillet: 148 calories, 2g fat (1g saturated fat), 42mg cholesterol, 358mg sodium, 5g carbohydrate (0 sugars, 0 fiber), 36g protein. Diabetic Exchanges: 6 lean meat, ½ starch.

IN-A-PINCH CHICKEN & SPINACH

Ingredients

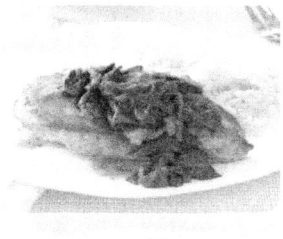

- 2 tsp olive oi
- 1 cup salsa
- 1 package (6 ounces) fresh baby spinach
- 1 tsp butter
- 4 boneless skinless chicken breast halves (6 ounces each)

Directions

1. Using a meat mallet, pound the chicken to a 12-inch thickness. Heat the oil and butter in a large skillet on a medium heat. Cook for 5-6 minutes on each side, or until the chicken is no longer pink then remove from the oven and keep warm.
2. Add spinach and salsa to pan and cook, stirring occasionally, for 3-4 minutes, or until spinach is wilted. Serve alongside chicken.

Nutrition Facts

1 chicken breast half with 1/3 cup spinach mixture: 182 calories, 12g fat (4g saturated fat), 102mg cholesterol, 176mg sodium, 6g carbohydrate (2g sugars, 1g fiber), 29g protein. Diabetic Exchanges: 5 lean meat, 2 fat, 1 vegetable.

SKILLET BEEF AND POTATOES

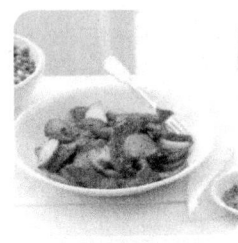

Ingredients

- 1/3 cup water
- 2 tsp garlic pepper blend
- 1-1/2 tsp minced fresh rosemary
- ½ tsp salt
- ½ cup chopped onion
- 3 tsp olive oil, divided
- 1-1/2 pounds red potatoes (about 5 medium), halved and cut into ¼-inch slices
- 1 pound beef top sirloin steak, cut into thin strips

Directions

1. In a microwave-safe dish, combine potatoes, water, and salt; microwave on high, covered, for 7-9 minutes, or until potatoes are tender. Drain.
2. Meanwhile, combine the beef, onion, 2 tablespoons oil, and pepper blend in a mixing bowl. Pre heat a large skillet to medium-high. Cook and stir until half of the meat mixture is browned, about 1-2 minutes. Remove the beef mixture from the pan and repeat with the remaining beef mixture.
3. Heat the remaining oil in a clean skillet over medium-high heat. Cook, stirring periodically, until potatoes are lightly browned, about 4-5 minutes. Heat through the beef mixture. Rosemary should be sprinkled on top.

Nutrition Facts

1-1/2 cups: 267 calories, 16g fat (5g saturated fat), 58mg cholesterol, 397mg sodium, 23g carbohydrate (2g sugars, 2g fiber), 23g protein. Diabetic Exchanges: 3 lean meat, 2 fat, 1 starch.

CHICKEN VEGGIE PACKETS

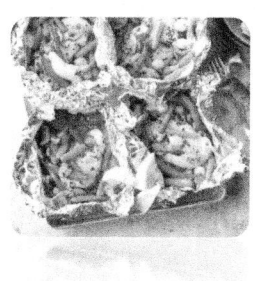

Ingredients

- 1-1/2 cups fresh baby carrots
- Lemon wedges, optional
- 1 cup pearl onions
- 3 tsp minced fresh thyme
- ½ tsp salt, optional
- 4 boneless skinless chicken breast halves (4 ounces each)
- 1/2 cup julienned sweet red pepper
- ½ pound sliced fresh mushrooms
- 1/4 tsp pepper

Directions

1. Preheat the oven to 375 degrees Fahrenheit. Flatten chicken breasts to a 1/2-inch thickness. Place each of them on a sheet of heavy-duty foil of equal thickness (about 12 in. square). Over the chicken,

layer the mushrooms, carrots, onions, and red pepper; season with pepper, thyme, and salt, if preferred.
2. Seal the foil tightly around the chicken and vegetables. Place the cookies on a baking pan. Cook for about 20 minutes, or until the chicken juices flow clear. Serve with lemon wedges if preferred.

Nutrition Facts

1 serving: 165 calories, 4g fat (1g saturated fat), 57mg cholesterol, 102mg sodium, 12g carbohydrate (6g sugars, 2g fiber), 24g protein. Diabetic Exchanges: 3 lean meat, 2 vegetable.

POACHED EGGS WITH TARRAGON ASPARAGUS

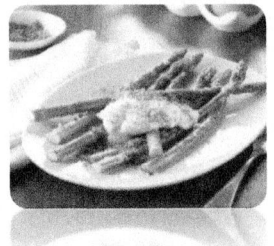

Ingredients

- 1 tsp olive oil
- ½ tsp salt
- ¼ tsp pepper
- 4 large eggs
- ¼ cup seasoned bread crumbs
- 1 tsp minced fresh tarragon
- 1-pound fresh asparagus, trimmed
- 1 tsp butter
- 1 garlic clove, minced

Directions

1. Fill a large skillet with 3 inches of water and allow to boil then add asparagus Cook, uncovered, for 2-4 minutes, or until asparagus is brilliant green. Remove the asparagus and immerse it in ice water right away. Drain and dry thoroughly.
2. Heat the oil in a separate large skillet over medium heat. Cook and stir for 1 minute after adding the garlic. Add the asparagus, tarragon, salt, and pepper; sauté for 2-3 minutes, stirring periodically, until crisp-tender. Remove from pan and set aside to keep heated. Heat the butter in the same skillet over medium heat. Cook and whisk for 1-2 minutes, or until bread crumbs are toasty. Turn off the heat
3. Pour 2-3 inches of fresh water into the skillet where the asparagus was cooked. Bring to a boil, then reduce to a low heat and keep at a soft simmer. Break cold eggs into a tiny bowl one at a time, bringing bowl close to water's surface and slipping egg into water.
4. Cook eggs for 3-4 minutes, uncovered, or until whites are completely set and yolks are thickening but not hard. Lift the eggs out of the water with a slotted spoon and serve over asparagus. Toss with toasted bread crumbs before serving.

Nutrition Facts

1 serving: 172 calories, 9g fat (4g saturated fat), 142mg cholesterol, 483mg sodium, 7g carbohydrate (2g sugars, 1g fiber), 8g protein. Diabetic Exchanges: 1-1/2 fat, 1 vegetable, 1 medium-fat meat

TURKEY CURRY

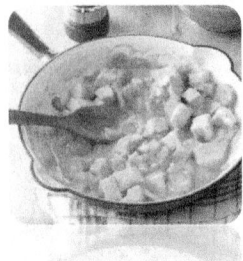

Ingredients

- 1 cup fat-free milk
- Hot cooked rice, optional
- 2 tsp cornstarch
- ¾ cup reduced-sodium chicken broth
- ½ cup sliced carrots
- 1 cup sliced celery
- 1 to 4 tsp curry powder
- 2 tsp dried minced onion
- 2 cups diced cooked turkey or chicken
- ½ tsp garlic powder

Directions

1. Spray a skillet lightly with cooking spray and cook celery and carrots until tender. Mix 1/4 cup milk and cornstarch in a bowl until smooth. Mix in the remaining milk and broth until smooth.
2. Pour the sauce all over the vegetables. Bring to a boil, then cook, stirring constantly, for 2 minutes, or until the sauce has thickened. Heat through the turkey, onion, garlic powder, and curry powder, stirring occasionally. If you want, you can serve it with rice.

Nutrition Facts

1 cup (calculated without rice): 172 calories, 3g fat (1g saturated fat), 72mg cholesterol, 235mg sodium, 12g

carbohydrate (5g sugars, 1g fiber), 24g protein. Diabetic Exchanges: 2 starch, 3 lean meat.

SEASONED TILAPIA FILLETS

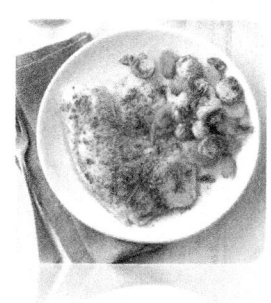

Ingredients

- 1 tsp butter, melted
- ½ tsp dried parsley flakes
- ¼ tsp paprika
- Dash garlic powder
- 1/8 tsp pepper
- ¼ tsp dried thyme
- 2 tilapia fillets (6 ounces each)
- 1/8 tsp onion powder
- 1 tsp Montreal steak seasoning
- 1/8 tsp salt

Directions

1. Pre- heat the oven to 425 degrees. Drizzle fish with butter in a buttered 11x7-inch baking dish. Mix the remaining ingredients in a small dish, sprinkle over fillets.
2. 2.Cover and bake for 10 minutes, uncover and bake for 5-8 minutes or until the fish flakes easily with a fork.

Nutrition Facts

1 fillet: 175 calories, 5g fat (5g saturated fat), 58mg cholesterol, 547mg sodium, 1g carbohydrate (0 sugars, 0 fiber), 32g protein. Diabetic Exchanges: 5 lean meat, 1-1/2 fat.

CHICKEN VEGGIE SKILLET

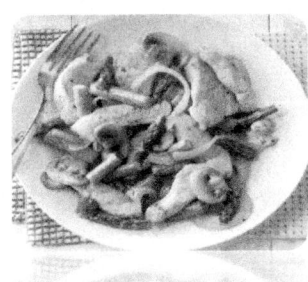

Ingredients

- 1-1/2 pounds boneless skinless chicken breasts, cut into ½-inch strips
- ½ tsp salt
- ¼ tsp pepper
- 1-pound fresh asparagus, trimmed and cut into 1-inch pieces
- 1 small onion, halved and sliced
- 6 tsp olive oil, divided
- ½ cup sherry or chicken stock
- ½ pound sliced fresh mushrooms
- 2 garlic cloves, minced
- 2 tsp cold butter, cubed

Directions

1. Season the chicken with pinch of salt and pepper.1 teaspoon oil, heated in a large skillet over medium-high heat Cook and stir for 3-4 minutes, or until the chicken is no longer pink. Repeat with the remaining chicken and 1 teaspoon oil.
2. Heat 2 teaspoons oil in the same pan, then add mushroom and onion cook and stir for 2-3 minutes, or until mushrooms and onion are soft. Cook for a further minute after adding the garlic. Toss in with the chicken.
3. In the same pan, heat the remaining oil. Cook for 2-3 minutes or until asparagus is crisp-tender, then add the chicken and mushrooms.
4. Stir in sherry to release browned pieces from the bottom of the pan. Bring to a boil, then reduce to 2 tablespoons of liquid by cooking for 1-2 minutes. Return the chicken and vegetables to the pan and heat until hot. Remove from heat and add 1 tablespoon of butter at a time.

Nutrition Facts

1 cup: 185 calories, 12g fat (4g saturated fat), 67mg cholesterol, 264mg sodium, 6g carbohydrate (3g sugars, 2g fiber), 26g protein. Diabetic Exchanges: 3 lean meat, 2 fat, 1 vegetable.

BAKED COD PICCATA WITH ASPARAGUS

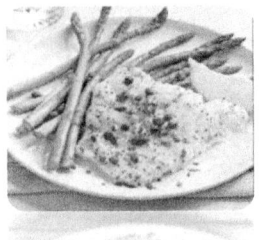

Ingredients

- 1 tsp salt-free lemon-pepper seasoning
- ¼ cup water
- Minced fresh parsley, optional
- ½ tsp garlic powder
- 1 pound cod fillet, cut into 4 pieces
- 2 tsp lemon juice
- 2 tsp butter, cubed
- 2 tsp capers
- 1-pound fresh asparagus, trimmed

Directions

1. Arrange asparagus in an 11x7-inch baking dish that hasn't been oiled. Add water to the baking dish. Arrange the cod on top of the asparagus. Lemon juice, lemon pepper, and garlic powder are sprinkled over top. Spread butter on top and top with capers.
2. Bake, uncovered, at 400° for 12-15 minutes, or until fish flakes easily with a fork and asparagus is tender, sprinkle with parsley if you desire.

Nutrition Facts

1 serving: 135 calories, 6g fat (4g saturated fat), 48mg cholesterol, 182mg sodium, 3g carbohydrate (1g sugars, 1g fiber), 23g protein. Diabetic Exchanges: 3 lean meat, 1 fat.

STIR-FRY RICE BOWL

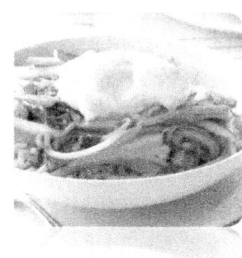

Ingredients

- 1 medium zucchini, julienned
- 1 cup bean sprouts
- 1 cup fresh baby spinach
- 1 tsp canola oil
- 1 tsp water
- ½ cup sliced baby portobello mushrooms
- 1 tsp sesame oil
- 1 tsp chili garlic sauce
- 1 tsp reduced-sodium soy sauce
- 4 large eggs
- 2 medium carrots, julienned
- 3 cups hot cooked brown rice

Directions

1. Heat canola oil in a large skillet over medium high heat. Cook and stir the carrots, zucchini, and mushrooms for 3-5 minutes, or until the carrots are crisp-tender. Cook and mix in the bean sprouts, spinach, water, soy sauce, and chili sauce until the spinach has wilted. Remove from the heat and set aside to keep warm.
2. Put 2–3 inches in a big skillet with high edges filled with water Bring to a boil, then reduce to a low heat and keep at a soft simmer. 1 at a time, crack cold eggs into a small dish; holding bowl close to water's surface, slip egg into water.
3. Cook for 3-5 minutes, uncovered, or until the whites are completely set and the yolks are thickening but not hard. Remove the eggs from the water using a slotted spoon.
4. Arrange the rice in bowls and top with the vegetables. Spray sesame oil on top. A poached egg should be placed on top of each plate

Nutrition Facts

1 serving: 269 calories, 12g fat (2g saturated fat), 147mg cholesterol, 364mg sodium, 40g carbohydrate (4g sugars, 4g fiber), 13g protein. Diabetic Exchanges: 2 starch, 2 medium-fat meat, 1 vegetable, 1 fat.

PEPPER STEAK WITH SQUASH

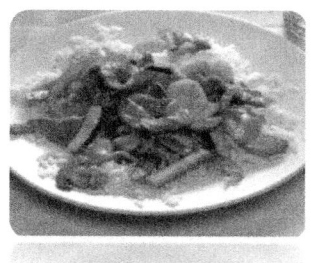

Ingredients

- 2 tsp canola oil, divided
- 1 can (14-1/2 ounces) reduced-sodium beef broth
- 1 beef flank steak (1 pound), cut into thin strips
- 1 medium sweet red pepper, cut into thin strips
- 1 cup sliced fresh mushrooms
- Hot cooked rice
- 3 tsp cornstarch
- 3 garlic cloves, minced
- 1 cup fresh snow peas
- 2 tsp reduced-sodium soy sauce
- 1 small onion, cut into thin strips
- 1 can (8 ounces) sliced water chestnuts, drained
- 2 medium zucchinis, cut into thin strips
- 1 medium green pepper, cut into thin strips

Directions

1. Whisk together the broth, soy sauce, and cornstarch until smooth then remove and keep aside.
2. Heat 1 tablespoon oil in a large skillet over medium heat. Stir-fry the meat for 2-3 minutes, or until it is no longer pink. Remove the pan from the heat.
3. Heat the remaining oil inside the same skillet. Peppers should be stir-fried for around 2 minutes. Cook and stir for another 2 minutes after adding the zucchini, onion, and garlic, snow peas, mushrooms,

and water chestnuts are all good additions. Stir fry for another 2 minutes, or until crisp-tender.
4. Add the cornstarch mixture to the pan and stir to mix. Bring to a boil, then cook and stir for 1-2 minutes, or until the sauce has thickened. Return the steak to the skillet and finish cooking it Serve with rice.

Nutrition Facts

1-1/2 cups stir-fry (calculated without rice): 217 calories, 9g fat (3g saturated fat), 38mg cholesterol, 353mg sodium, 18g carbohydrate (6g sugars, 4g fiber), 18g protein. Diabetic Exchanges: 2 lean meat, 1 vegetable, ½ starch.

CURRY TURKEY STIR-FRY

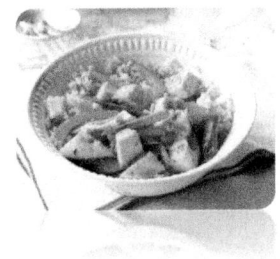

Ingredients

- 2 tsp reduced-sodium soy sauce
- 1/8 tsp crushed red pepper flakes, optional
- 1 tsp curry powder
- ½ tsp cornstarch
- 2 cups hot cooked brown rice
- 2 cups cubed cooked turkey breast

- 1 large sweet red pepper, julienned
- 1 tsp sesame or canola oil
- 1 garlic clove, minced
- 1 tsp minced fresh cilantro
- 1 tsp canola oil
- 1 tsp honey
- 3 green onions, cut into 2-inch pieces

Directions

1. Combine the ingredients and chili flakes (if needed) in a mixing bowl. Use 1 tablespoon of rapeseed oil in a large frying pan over medium-high heat to fry the red peppers until crisp, about 2 minutes. Add onions and cook for 1-2 minutes, or until tender.
2. Add the cornstarch mixture to the pot and stir to combine. Bring to a boil, then cook and stir for 1-2 minutes, or until the sauce thickens. Heat the turkey thoroughly by stirring. Serve with rice

Nutrition Facts

¾ cup turkey mixture with ½ cup rice: 257 calories, 7g fat (1g saturated fat), 56mg cholesterol, 268mg sodium, 21g carbohydrate (7g sugars, 3g fiber), 25g protein. Diabetic Exchanges: 3 lean meat, 2 starch, 1 fat.

MEDITERRANEAN TILAPIA

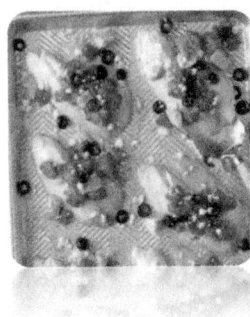

Ingredients

- 1 cup canned Italian diced tomatoes
- 6 tilapia fillets (6 ounces each)
- ½ cup sliced ripe olives
- ½ cup crumbled feta cheese
- ½ cup water-packed artichoke hearts, chopped

Directions

Pre- heat the oven to 400 degrees then Coat a 15x10x1-inch baking sheet with cooking spray and place the fillets inside, tomatoes, artichoke hearts, olives, and cheese can be added on the top. Cover and bake for 15-20 minutes, or until fish flakes readily with a fork.

Nutrition Facts

1 fillet: 159 calories, 5g fat (2g saturated fat), 68mg cholesterol, 463mg sodium, 6g carbohydrate (2g sugars, 1g fiber), 35g protein. Diabetic exchanges: 5 lean meat, ½ fat.

ROSEMARY GARLIC SHRIMP

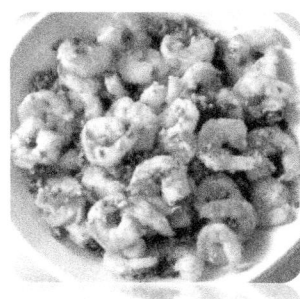

Ingredients

- 1-1/4 cups chicken or vegetable broth
- 3 tsp chopped ripe olives
- 1 tsp paprika
- ¼ to ½ tsp pepper
- 1 tsp minced fresh rosemary or 1 teaspoon dried rosemary, crushed
- 1 small cayenne or other fresh red chili pepper, finely chopped
- ½ teaspoon salt
- 2 pounds uncooked shrimp (31-40 per pound), peeled and deveined
- 4 garlic cloves, minced
- 2 tsp lemon juice
- 2 tsp Worcestershire sauce

Directions

1. Bring all of the ingredients, except the shrimp, to a boil in a large skillet. Cook until the liquid has been reduced by half, uncovered.
2. Add the shrimp and bring to a boil. Reduce heat to low and cook, uncovered, for 3-4 minutes, or until shrimp turn pink, turning occasionally.

Nutrition Facts

½ cup: 130 calories, 4g fat (0 saturated fat), 128mg cholesterol, 458mg sodium, 3g carbohydrate (1g sugars, 0 fiber), 18g protein. Diabetic Exchanges: 3 lean meat.

STUFFED-OLIVE COD

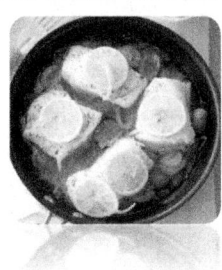

Ingredients

- 1 tsp dried oregano
- 1/3 cup garlic-stuffed olives, halved
- ¼ tsp salt
- 1 shallot, thinly sliced
- 2 tsp olive juice
- 2 tsp water
- 4 cod fillets (6 ounces each)
- 1 medium lemon, thinly sliced

Directions

1. Spray a large nonstick skillet with cooking spray and place the fillets in it. Season with salt and oregano, then top with lemon and shallot.
2. Arrange olives around the fish and cover with water and olive juice. Bring the water to a boil. Reduce

heat to low and simmer for 8-10 minutes, covered, or until fish flakes easily with a fork.

Nutrition Facts

1 fillet: 143 calories, 4g fat (0 saturated fat), 58mg cholesterol, 598mg sodium, 5g carbohydrate (1g sugars, 0 fiber), 26g protein. Diabetic Exchanges: 4 lean meat.

LEMON-PEPPER TILAPIA WITH MUSHROOMS

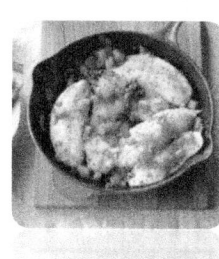

Ingredients

- 2 Tsp butter
- 4 tilapia fillets (6 ounces each)
- ¾ tsp lemon-pepper seasoning, divided
- 3 garlic cloves, minced
- ¼ tsp paprika
- 3 green onions, thinly sliced
- 1/8 tsp cayenne pepper
- 1 medium tomato, chopped
- ½ pound sliced fresh mushrooms

Directions

1. Melt butter in a 12- inch skillet over medium heat. Cook and stir for 3-5 minutes, or until mushrooms and 1/4 tsp lemon pepper are soft. Cook for another 30 seconds after adding the garlic.
2. Arrange the fillets on top of the mushrooms and season with paprika, cayenne, and the remaining lemon pepper. Cook for 5-7 minutes, covered, or until the salmon flakes easily with a fork. Tomato and green onions go on top.

Nutrition Facts

1 fillet: 159 calories, 7g fat (4g saturated fat), 102mg cholesterol, 165mg sodium, 5g carbohydrate (3g sugars, 1g fiber), 32g protein. Diabetic Exchanges: 4 lean meat, 1-1/2 fat.

CHICKEN SAUSAGES WITH POLENTA

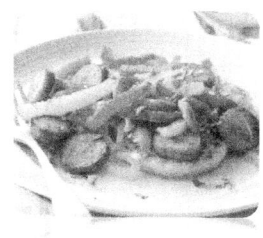

Ingredients

- 4 tsp olive oil, divided
- 1 tube (1 pound) polenta, cut into ½-inch slices
- 1 medium onion, thinly sliced
- 1 package (12 ounces) fully cooked Italian chicken sausage links, thinly sliced
- 1 tsp minced fresh basil
- ¼ cup grated Parmesan cheese
- 1 each medium green, sweet red and yellow peppers, thinly sliced

Directions

1. 2 teaspoons oil, heated in a large nonstick skillet over medium heat, cook polenta for 8-10 minutes on each side or until golden brown. Keep warm.
2. Heat the remaining oil in a large skillet over medium high heat. Cook, stirring frequently until the peppers and onion are soft. Remove the pan from the heat.
3. In the same pan, cook and stir sausages for 4-5 minutes, or until browned. Return the pepper mixture to the pan and heat until hot. Serve with polenta, cheese, and basil on top

Nutrition Facts

2/3 cup sausage mixture with 2 slices polenta: 184 calories, 9g fat (2g saturated fat), 42mg cholesterol, 628mg sodium, 17g carbohydrate (4g sugars, 2g fiber), 14g protein. Diabetic Exchanges: 2 lean meat, 1 starch, 1 vegetable, ½ fat.

SALMON WITH SPINACH & WHITE BEANS

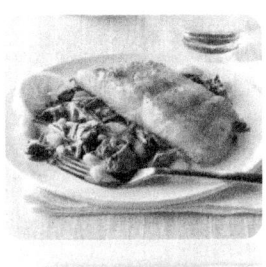

Ingredients

- 4 salmon fillets (4 ounces each)
- Lemon wedges
- 1 tsp seafood seasoning
- ¼ tsp salt
- 1 package (8 ounces) fresh spinach
- 1 garlic clove, minced
- 2 tsp plus 1 tablespoon olive oil, divided
- 1 can (15 ounces) cannellini beans, rinsed and drained
- ¼ tsp pepper

Directions

1. Pre heat the oven to broil, 2 teaspoons oil, 2 teaspoons seafood seasoning. Place on a greased

broiler pan rack, broil 5-6 inches 7-8 minutes from heat or until salmon just begins to flake easily with a fork.
2. Meanwhile, heat the remaining oil in a large skillet over medium heat, let cook 15-30 seconds or until garlic is aromatic. Stir in the beans, salt, and pepper to coat them in garlic oil. Stir in the spinach and cook until it is wilted. Serve the salmon with the spinach combination and lemon wedges on the side.

Nutrition Facts

1 fillet with ½ cup spinach mixture: 247 calories, 18g fat (4g saturated fat), 48mg cholesterol, 457mg sodium, 16g carbohydrate (0 sugars, 5g fiber), 26g protein. Diabetic Exchanges: 3 lean meat, 2 vegetable, 2 fat, ½ starch.

GINGER VEGGIE BROWN RICE PASTA

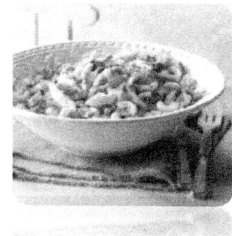

Ingredients

- 2 cups uncooked brown rice elbow pasta
- ½ small red onion, sliced
- 2 tsp ginger paste
- 2 tsp garlic paste
- 1-1/2 cups chopped fresh Brussels sprouts
- ½ cup chopped red cabbage

- ½ cup shredded carrots
- 1 tsp coconut oil
- ½ medium sweet red pepper, chopped
- ½ teaspoon salt
- 2 green onions, chopped
- ¼ tsp ground ancho chile pepper
- ¼ tsp coarsely ground pepper
- 1 rotisserie chicken, skin removed, shredded

Directions

1. Cook pasta as directed on the package in a Dutch oven.
2. In the meantime, melt coconut oil in a large skillet over medium heat. Sauté for 2 minutes with the red onion, ginger, and garlic paste. Cook until vegetables are crisp-tender, about 4-6 minutes, after adding the following first 7 ingredients. Return the chicken to the pan and heat until it is fully cooked.
3. 1 cup pasta water should be set aside after draining the noodles. Back in the Dutch oven, add the spaghetti. Toss in the vegetable mixture, being careful not to overcook the noodles. Before serving, top with chopped green onions.

Nutrition Facts

1 cup: 243 calories, 6g fat (2g saturated fat), 55mg cholesterol, 357mg sodium, 29g carbohydrate (3g sugars, 3g fiber), 24g protein. Diabetic Exchanges: 3 lean meat, 2 starch, 2 fat.

SPICY TURKEY LETTUCE WRAPS

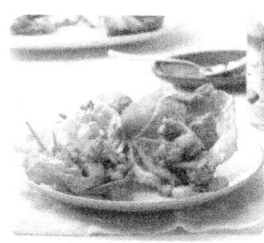

Ingredients

- ¼ cup chopped onion
- 1/2 cup chopped peeled jicama or celery
- 2 tsp reduced-sodium soy sauce
- ¼ cup julienned carrot
- ½ pound lean ground turkey
- 1/8 tsp cayenne pepper
- 2 tsp minced fresh gingerroot
- 1 garlic clove, minced
- 1/8 tsp pepper
- 6 Bibb lettuce leaves
- Hot mustard, optional

Directions

1. Cook turkey, jicama, and onion in a large skillet over medium heat until no longer pink, about 4-6 minutes. Soy sauce, ginger, garlic, and peppers should all be added at this point. Cook and stir for 1-2 minutes, or until liquid has been absorbed.
2. Place lettuce on top of the dish. Garnish with mustard if desired.

Nutrition Facts

2 wraps: 215calories, 7g fat (3g saturated fat), 74mg cholesterol, 562mg sodium, 9g carbohydrate (2g sugars,

4g fiber), 22g protein. Diabetic Exchanges: 3 lean meat, 1 vegetable.

SPICED SALMON

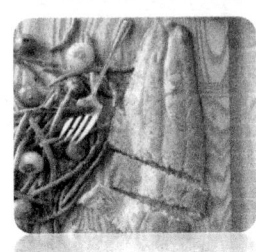

Ingredients

- 2 tsp packed brown sugar
- 1 tsp olive oil
- ½ tsp paprika
- ½ tsp garlic powder
- ½ tsp ground mustard
- 1 tsp butter, melted
- Dash cayenne pepper
- ½ tsp pepper
- Dash salt
- Dash dried tarragon
- 1 tsp soy sauce
- ¼ tsp dill weed
- 1 salmon fillet (2 pounds)

Directions

1. Combine all ingredients except the salmon and brush over it.
2. Place the salmon, skin side down, on a lightly oiled grill rack or baking sheet. Grill, covered, over medium heat or broil 4 inches from heat for 10-15

minutes, or until salmon just begins to flake easily with a fork.

Nutrition Facts

3 ounces cooked salmon: 273 calories, 12g fat (5g saturated fat), 65mg cholesterol, 320mg sodium, 6g carbohydrate (6g sugars, 0 fiber), 25g protein. Diabetic Exchanges: 3 lean meat, 1-1/2 fat.

CHICKEN & GOAT CHEESE SKILLET

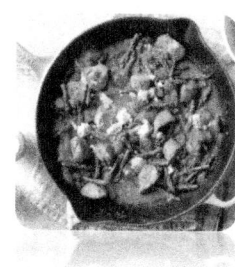

Ingredients

- ½ pound boneless skinless chicken breasts, cut into 1-inch pieces
- ¼ tsp salt
- 1/8 tsp pepper
- Additional goat cheese, optional
- 3 plum tomatoes, chopped
- 2 tsp olive oil
- 1 garlic clove, minced
- 3 tsp 2% milk
- 2 tsp herbed fresh goat cheese, crumbled
- Hot cooked rice or pasta
- 1 cup cut fresh asparagus (1-inch pieces)

Directions

1. sprinkle the chicken with salt and pepper before serving. Heat oil in a large skillet over medium-high heat and cook chicken until no longer pink, about 4-6 minutes. Remove from the pan and set aside to keep heated.
2. Cook and stir asparagus in a skillet over medium-high heat for 1 minutes. Cook and stir for 30 seconds after adding the garlic, Cook, covered, over medium heat until tomatoes, milk, and 2 tablespoons cheese begin to melt, about 2-3 minutes then add the chicken and stir well. Serve alongside rice. If desired additional cheese can be added.

Nutrition Facts

1-1/2 cups chicken mixture: 261 calories, 10g fat (4g saturated fat), 64mg cholesterol, 367mg sodium, 8g carbohydrate (4g sugars, 3g fiber), 24g protein. Diabetic Exchanges: 4 lean meat, 2 fat, 1 vegetable.

GARLIC-MUSHROOM TURKEY SLICES

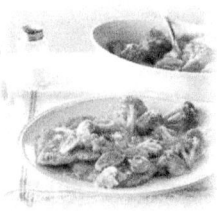

Ingredients

- ½ cup all-purpose flour
- ½ tsp dried oregano
- 2 garlic cloves, minced

- ¾ cup reduced-sodium chicken broth
- ¾ tsp salt, divided
- ½ pound sliced fresh mushrooms
- ¼ tsp pepper, divided
- 1 tsp olive oil
- ½ tsp paprika
- ¼ cup dry white wine or additional broth
- 1 package (17.6 ounces) turkey breast cutlets

Directions

1. Combine flour, oregano, paprika, 1/2 teaspoon salt, and 1/8 teaspoon pepper in a large shallow dish. Dip cutlets in flour mixture to cover both sides; brush off excess.
2. Heat oil in a large nonstick skillet over medium heat. Cook turkey in batches for 1-2 minutes per side or until no longer pink, remove from pan.
3. Stir in the remaining salt and pepper to the skillet with the remaining ingredients. Cook, stirring occasionally, for 4-6 minutes, or until mushrooms are soft. Return the turkey to the pan and cook through, turning to coat all sides.

Nutrition Facts

1 serving: 118 calories, 4g fat (1g saturated fat), 77mg cholesterol, 426mg sodium, 8g carbohydrate (1g sugars, 1g fiber), 32g protein. Diabetic Exchanges: 3 lean meat, ½ starch, ½ fat.

GRILLED CHICKEN CHOPPED SALAD

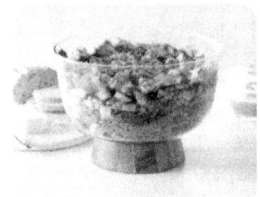

Ingredients

- 1 pound chicken tenderloins
- 1 medium cucumber, chopped
- 6 tsp zesty Italian salad dressing, divided
- Additional salad dressing, optional
- 1 medium red onion, quartered
- 2 medium ears sweet corn, husks removed
- 1 bunch romaine, chopped
- 2 medium zucchinis, quartered lengthwise

Directions

1. Toss the chicken with 4 tablespoons of the dressing in a mixing bowl. Brush the remaining 2 tablespoons of dressing over the zucchini and onion.
2. Close the cover and place the corn, zucchini, and onion on a grill rack over medium heat. Grill the zucchini and onions for 2-3 minutes on each side, or until they are soft. Grill corn for 10-12 minutes, turning once or twice, until tender.
3. Drain the chicken and toss out the marinade. Cover and grill the chicken for 3-4 minutes on each side over medium heat, or until no longer pink.
4. Remove the corn off the cobs and cut the zucchini, onion, and chicken into bite-size pieces. In a 3-quart baking dish, combine the flour, sugar, and salt. Layer romaine, cucumber, grilled veggies, and chicken in a

trifle dish or other glass bowl. Serve with extra dressing if desired.

Nutrition Facts

3 cups: 226 calories, 6g fat (0 saturated fat), 46mg cholesterol, 176mg sodium, 21g carbohydrate (8g sugars, 5g fiber), 32g protein. Diabetic Exchanges: 3 lean meat, 2 vegetable, ½ starch, ½ fat.

NAKED FISH TACOS

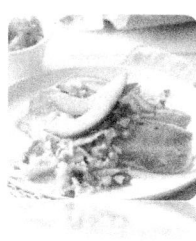

Ingredients

- 1 cup coleslaw mix
- ½ medium ripe avocado, peeled and sliced
- ½ tsp ground cumin
- 1/4 cup chopped fresh cilantro
- 1 green onion, sliced
- 1 tsp chopped seeded jalapeno pepper
- 4 tsp canola oil, divided
- 2 tsp lime juice
- ½ tsp salt, divided
- 1/4 tsp pepper, divided
- 2 tilapia fillets (6 ounces each)

Directions

1. Toss the first four ingredients with 2 tablespoons oil, lime juice, cumin, 1/4 teaspoon salt, and 1/8 teaspoon pepper in a mixing bowl. Refrigerate until ready to be served.
2. Using paper towels, pat the fillets dry and season with the remaining salt and pepper then cook tilapia in remaining oil in a large nonstick skillet over medium-high heat until it just begins to flake easily with a fork, 3-4 minutes each side. Serve with slaw and avocado on top

Nutrition Facts

1 serving: 246 calories, 12g fat (2g saturated fat), 78mg cholesterol, 663mg sodium, 6g carbohydrate (1g sugars, 3g fiber), 26g protein. Diabetic Exchanges: 5 lean meat, 3 fat, 1 vegetable.

TILAPIA WITH CITRUS SAUCE

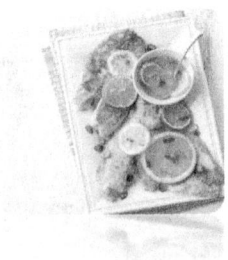

Ingredients

- ½ cup 2% milk
- ½ cup all-purpose flour
- ½ tsp salt
- ½ tsp pepper

- 2 green onions, finely chopped
- 4 tilapia fillets (4 ounces each)
- Olive oil-flavored cooking spray
- 3 tsp lime juice
- 3 garlic cloves, minced
- 2 green onions, finely chopped
- ½ medium lime, sliced
- 1 tsp butter
- 2 tsp orange juice
- 2 tsp olive oil
- ½ small lemon, sliced
- ½ small navel orange, sliced
- 3 tsp lemon juice

Directions

1. Fill a shallow bowl halfway with milk. Whisk the flour, salt, and pepper in a small bowl, after dipping the fish in the milk, coat it in the flour mixture.
2. cover the fillets in cooking spray then cook fish for 3-4 minutes on each side in a large nonstick skillet over medium-high heat or until it flakes easily with a fork then remove it from the oven and keep warm.
3. Sauté garlic in butter and oil for 1 minute in the same pan cook for 1 minute further after adding the lemon, lime, and orange slices, liquids, and onions. Serve alongside seafood.

Nutrition Facts.

1 fillet with ¼ cup sauce: 153calories, 7g fat (5g saturated fat), 69mg cholesterol, 129mg sodium, 11g

carbohydrate (3g sugars, 1g fiber), 24g protein. Diabetic Exchanges: 3 lean meat, 1 fat, ½ fruit.

CHICKEN WITH FIRE-ROASTED TOMATOES

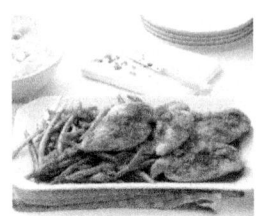

Ingredients

- ½ tsp salt
- 1/8 tsp crushed red pepper flakes, optional
- ¼ tsp Italian seasoning
- ¼ tsp pepper
- 1 tsp olive oil
- 1 can (14-1/2 ounces) fire-roasted diced tomatoes, undrained
- ¾ pound fresh green beans, trimmed
- 2 tsp water
- Hot cooked pasta, optional
- 2 tsp salt-free garlic herb seasoning blend
- 1 tsp butter
- 4 boneless skinless chicken breast halves (6 ounces each)

Directions

1. Combine the seasoning ingredients and season both sides of the chicken breasts then heat the oil in a

large skillet over medium heat. Both sides of the chicken should be browned. Bring to a boil with the tomatoes. Reduce heat to low; cover and cook for 10-12 minutes, or until a thermometer inserted in the chicken registers 165 degrees.
2. Meanwhile, combine green beans and water in a 2-quart microwave-safe dish, microwave, covered, on high for 3-4 minutes or until tender. Drain.
3. Remove the chicken from the skillet and keep it aside to keep warm. Toss the tomato combination with the butter and beans. Serve with chicken and pasta, if desired

Nutrition Facts

1 chicken breast half with 1 cup bean mixture: 264 calories, 10g fat (3g saturated fat), 97mg cholesterol, 581mg sodium, 14g carbohydrate (5g sugars, 4g fiber), 34g protein. Diabetic Exchanges: 5 lean meat, 1 vegetable, 1 fat.

COD WITH BACON & BALSAMIC TOMATOES

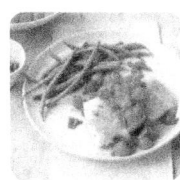

Ingredients

- 4 cod fillets (5 ounces each)
- 4 center-cut bacon strips, chopped
- ½ tsp salt
- 2 tsp balsamic vinegar

- ¼ tsp pepper
- 2 cups grape tomatoes, halved

Directions

1. Cook bacon, stirring occasionally, in a large skillet over medium heat until crisp. Drain on paper towels using a slotted spoon.
2. Salt and pepper the fillets. Cook the fillets in the bacon drippings for 4-6 minutes on each side over medium-high heat, or until the fish flakes easily with a fork and remove from the heat and put aside.
3. Add the tomatoes to the skillet and cook, stirring occasionally, for 2-4 minutes, or until softened. Reduce heat to low and stir in the vinegar and cook for another 1-2 minutes until sauce has thickened. Serve the cod with a tomato-bacon sauce.

Nutrition Facts

1 fillet with ¼ cup tomato mixture and 1 tablespoon bacon: 187 calories, 7g fat (2g saturated fat), 56mg cholesterol, 395mg sodium, 5g carbohydrate (4g sugars, 2g fiber), 24g protein. Diabetic Exchanges: 4 lean meat, 1 vegetable.

CILANTRO LIME SHRIMP

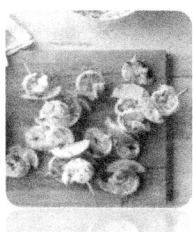

Ingredients

- 1/3 cup chopped fresh cilantro
- 1/3 cup lime juice
- ¼ tsp ground cumin
- 1 jalapeno pepper, seeded and minced
- 2 tsp olive oil
- 1-pound uncooked shrimp (16-20 per pound), peeled and deveined
- 3 garlic cloves, minced
- ¼ tsp salt
- 1-1/2 tsp grated lime zest
- ¼ tsp pepper
- Lime slices

Directions

1. Toss the shrimp with the first 9 ingredients. Allow 15 minutes to rest before serving.
2. Using 4 metal or soaked wooden skewers, thread shrimp and lime slices. Cover and grill for 2-4 minutes per side over medium heat, or until shrimp turn pink.

Nutrition Facts

1 kabob: 157 calories, 7g fat (1g saturated fat), 168mg cholesterol, 284mg sodium, 5g carbohydrate (1g sugars, 0

fiber), 16g protein. Diabetic Exchanges: 3 lean meat, 1-1/2 fat.

CRUNCHY TUNA SALAD WITH TOMATOES

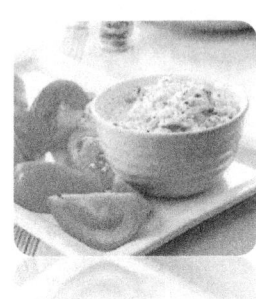

Ingredients

- 2/3 cup reduced-fat mayonnaise
- 1 tsp minced fresh parsley or ¼ teaspoon dried parsley flakes
- ½ cup chopped sweet onion
- 1 can (12 ounces) albacore white tuna in water, drained and flaked
- 4 medium tomatoes, cut into wedges
- ¾ tsp pepper
- 1 celery rib, chopped

Directions

In a mixing bowl, combine mayonnaise, onion, celery, parsley and pepper and Stir in tuna. Serve with tomato wedges.

Nutrition Facts

½ cup tuna salad with 1 tomato: 258 calories, 17g fat (4g saturated fat), 50mg cholesterol, 656mg sodium, 14g carbohydrate (6g sugars,4g fiber), 24g protein. Diabetic Exchanges: 3 lean meat, 2 fat, 1 vegetable.

PEPPERED TUNA KABOBS

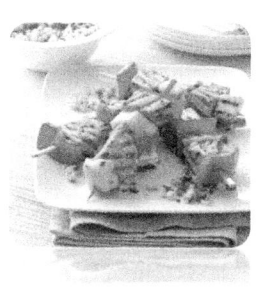

Ingredients

- ½ cup frozen corn, thawed
- 4 green onions, chopped
- 2 tsp coarsely chopped fresh parsley
- 2 tsp lime juice
- 2 large sweet red peppers, cut into 2x1-inch pieces
- 1 pound tuna steaks, cut into 1-inch cubes
- 1 tsp coarsely ground pepper
- 1 medium mango, peeled and cut into 1-inch cubes
- 1 jalapeno pepper, seeded and chopped

Directions

1. To make the salsa, combine the first five ingredients in a small bowl and set aside.
2. Season tuna with black pepper. Thread red peppers, tuna, and mango alternately on four metal or moistened wooden skewers.
3. Arrange the skewers on a grill rack that has been greased. Cook, covered, over medium heat, stirring periodically, for 10-12 minutes, or until tuna is

barely pink in the middle (medium-rare) and peppers are soft. Serve with a side of salsa.

Nutrition Facts

1 kabob: 179 calories, 4g fat (0 saturated fat), 49mg cholesterol, 52mg sodium, 18g carbohydrate (14g sugars, 4g fiber), 19g protein. Diabetic Exchanges: 3 lean meat, 1 starch.

CHICKEN & SPANISH CAULIFLOWER "RICE"

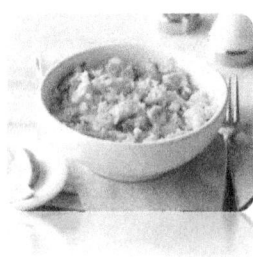

Ingredients

- ½ tsp salt
- ½ tsp pepper
- 1 tsp lime juice
- 1 tsp canola oil
- ¼ cup chopped fresh cilantro
- 1 large head cauliflower
- 1 medium green pepper, chopped
- 1 small onion, chopped
- 1-pound boneless skinless chicken breasts, cut into ½-inch cubes
- ½ cup tomato juice
- ¼ tsp ground cumin
- 1 garlic clove, minced

Directions

1. Peel and core the cauliflower, then cut it into 1-inch pieces. In a food processor, pulse cauliflower in batches until it resembles rice (do not overprocess).
2. Season the chicken with salt and pepper before serving. Heat the oil in a large skillet over medium-high heat and cook the chicken until it is nicely browned, about 5 minutes. Cook and stir for 3 minutes after adding the green pepper, onion, and garlic.
3. Add the tomato juice and cumin to the pot and bring to a boil. Cook, covered, over medium heat for 7-10 minutes, or until cauliflower is cooked, stirring occasionally. Add the cilantro and lime juice and mix well.

Nutrition Facts

1-1/2 cups: 234 calories, 6g fat (2g saturated fat), 65mg cholesterol, 347mg sodium, 16g carbohydrate (7g sugars, 6g fiber), 28g protein. Diabetic Exchanges: 3 lean meat, 1 starch, ½ fat.

CHERRY-CHICKEN LETTUCE WRAPS

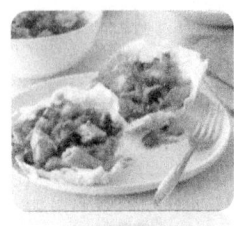

Ingredients

- 1 tsp ground ginger
- 1/4 tsp salt
- 1/4 tsp pepper
- ¾ pound boneless skinless chicken breasts, cut into ¾-inch cubes
- 2 tsp olive oil
- 1-1/2 cups shredded carrots
- 2 tsp reduced-sodium teriyaki sauce
- 1-1/4 cups coarsely chopped pitted fresh sweet cherries
- 1/3 cup coarsely chopped almonds
- 2 tsp rice vinegar
- 1 tsp honey
- 4 green onions, chopped
- 8 Bibb or Boston lettuce leaves

Directions

1. Season the chicken with salt and pepper and a dash of ginger. Heat the oil in a large nonstick skillet over medium- high heat and cook, stir for 3-5 minutes, or until the chicken is no longer pink.
2. Turn off the heat. Combine carrots, cherries, green onions, and almonds in a mixing bowl. Combine vinegar, teriyaki sauce, and honey in a small basin; stir into chicken mixture. Divide the filling among the lettuce leaves and fold the lettuce over the filling.

Nutrition Facts

2 filled lettuce wraps: 268 calories, 12g fat (1g saturated fat), 47mg cholesterol, 261mg sodium, 18g carbohydrate (16g sugars, 5g fiber), 18g protein. Diabetic Exchanges: 3 lean meat, 1 vegetable, ½ fruit, ½ fat.

PEPPER AND SALSA COD

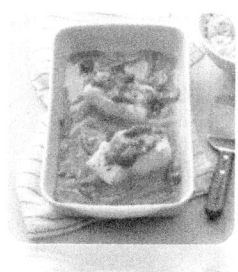

Ingredients

- 1 tsp olive oil
- 1/3 cup julienned green pepper
- ¼ tsp salt
- Dash pepper
- 1/3 cup julienned sweet red pepper
- 1/3 cup orange juice
- ¼ cup salsa
- Hot cooked rice
- 2 cod or haddock fillets (6 ounces each)

Directions

1. Pre heat the oven to 350 degrees. Brush the fillets on both sides with oil and arrange them in a greased 11x7-inch baking dish. Season to taste with salt and

pepper. Pour orange juice over the fish and serve with salsa and peppers on the side.
2. Bake, covered, for 17-20 minutes, or until fish just begins to flake easily with a fork. Serve with rice by the side

Nutrition Facts

1 serving: 159 calories, 4g fat (1g saturated fat), 58mg cholesterol, 486mg sodium, 8g carbohydrate (6g sugars, 1g fiber), 25g protein. Diabetic Exchanges: 4 lean meat, 1 vegetable, ½ fat.

SIMPLE GRILLED STEAK FAJITAS

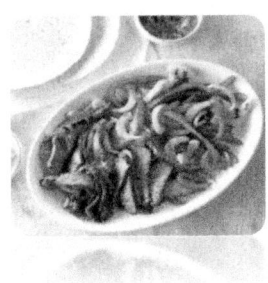

Ingredients

- 1 beef top sirloin steak (3/4 inch thick and 1 pound)
- 4 whole wheat tortillas (8 inches), warmed
- 1 large sweet onion, cut crosswise into ½-inch slices
- 1 medium sweet red pepper, halved
- 1 medium green pepper, halved
- Sliced avocado, optional
- Minced fresh cilantro, optional
- 1 tsp olive oil

- Lime wedges, optional
- 2 tsp fajita seasoning mix

Directions

1. Season the steak with the seasoning mix. Using a brush, coat the onion and peppers in oil.
2. Cook the steak and vegetables on a greased rack over medium direct heat, covered. 4-6 minutes each side or until meat reaches desired doneness (a thermometer should read 135° for medium-rare, 140° for medium, and 145° for medium-well) and veggies are soft, then you remove the grill from the heat. Allow 5 minutes for the steak to rest, covered, before slicing.
3. Slice the vegetables and steak into strips and place them in tortillas. Top with avocado and cilantro, if desired, then lime wedges to serve.

Nutrition Facts

1 serving: 296 calories, 14g fat (5g saturated fat), 47mg cholesterol, 686mg sodium, 36g carbohydrate (7g sugars, 6g fiber), 24g protein. Diabetic Exchanges: 3 lean meat, 2 starch, 1 vegetable, ½ fat.

TURKEY VERDE LETTUCE WRAPS

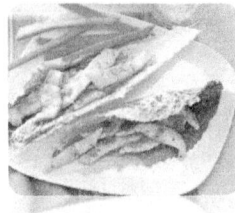

Ingredients

- 4 tsp olive oil
- 12 romaine leaves
- 1 Tsp garlic salt
- 1/4 tsp pepper
- 1 cup salsa Verde
- 2 packages (17.6 ounces each) turkey breast cutlets, cut into 1-inch strips

Directions

Combine the turkey, oil, garlic salt, and pepper in a large mixing basin, in a large skillet, heat the oil over medium-high heat. Cook and stir the turkey mixture in batches for 2-4 minutes, or until no longer pink. Return all of the turkey to the pan. Toss in the salsa and heat thoroughly. Serve on romaine lettuce.

Nutrition Facts

2 lettuce wraps: 274 calories, 3g fat (2g saturated fat), 106mg cholesterol, 579mg sodium, 4g carbohydrate (2g sugars, 3g fiber), 37g protein. Diabetic Exchanges: 5 lean meat, ½ fat.

GARLIC TILAPIA WITH SPICY KALE

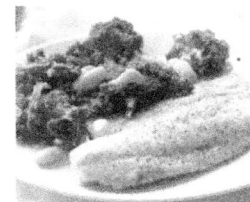

Ingredients

- 3 tsp olive oil, divided
- 4 tilapia fillets (6 ounces each)
- 1 bunch kale, trimmed and coarsely chopped (about 16 cups)
- 2 garlic cloves, minced
- ½ tsp crushed red pepper flakes
- 1 tsp fennel seed
- 1 can (15 ounces) cannellini beans, rinsed and drained
- 2/3 cup water
- ½ tsp salt
- ¾ tsp pepper, divided
- ½ tsp garlic salt

Directions

1. Heat 1 tablespoon oil in a 6-quart stockpot over medium heat. Cook and stir for 1 minute after adding the garlic, fennel, and pepper flakes. Bring the kale and water to a boil. Reduce to a low heat and cook, covered, for 10-12 minutes, or until the kale is soft.
2. In the meantime, season the tilapia with 12 teaspoon pepper and a pinch of garlic salt. Heat the remaining oil in a large skillet over medium heat. Cook the tilapia for 3-4 minutes on each side, or until it flakes easily with a fork.

3. Toss the kale with the beans, salt, and remaining pepper; heat through, stirring occasionally. Serve alongside tilapia

Nutrition Facts

1 fillet with 1 cup kale mixture: 287 calories, 14g fat (3g saturated fat), 83mg cholesterol, 645mg sodium, 23g carbohydrate (0 sugars, 6g fiber), 36g protein. Diabetic Exchanges: 5 lean meat, 2 fat, 1-1/2 starch.

GRILLED CHICKEN AND MANGO SKEWERS

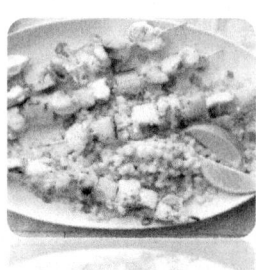

Ingredients

- Lime wedges, optional
- 1 tsp butter
- 1/3 cup plus 3 tablespoons sliced green onions, divided
- 1-pound boneless skinless chicken breasts, cut into 1-inch cubes
- ½ tsp salt
- 3 medium ears sweet corn
- 1 tsp extra virgin olive oil
- ¼ teaspoon pepper

- 1 medium mango, peeled and cut into 1-inch cubes

Directions

1. Remove the cobs of corn. Heat butter in a large skillet over medium-high heat, then sauté sliced corn for 5 minutes, or until crisp-tender. 1/3 cup green onions should be added at this point. Warmth is essential.
2. Season the chicken with salt and pepper before tossing it in the pan. Using 4 metal or soaked wooden skewers, alternate threading chicken and mango. Apply a layer of oil to the surface.
3. Cover and grill over medium heat or broil 4 inches from heat for 10-12 minutes, turning occasionally, until chicken is no longer pink.
4. Toss in the remaining green onions and serve with the corn mixture. Lime wedges can be added if desired.

Nutrition Facts

1 skewer with ½ cup corn mixture: 187 calories, 7g fat (4g saturated fat), 64mg cholesterol, 387mg sodium, 24g carbohydrate (18g sugars, 4g fiber), 27g protein. Diabetic Exchanges: 3 lean meat, 2 starch, 1-1/2 fat.

Printed in Great Britain
by Amazon